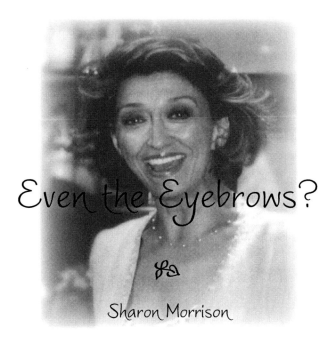

Even the Eyebrows?

Sharon Morrison

authorHOUSE®

AuthorHouse™ UK Ltd.
500 Avebury Boulevard
Central Milton Keynes, MK9 2BE
www.authorhouse.co.uk
Phone: 08001974150

First published by AuthorHouse 2/25/2009

ISBN: 978-1-4389-2334-5 (sc)

Printed in the United States of America
Bloomington, Indiana

This book is printed on acid-free paper.

For Leanne

Contents

૪ৈ

Foreword by Professor Gordon McVie

꿇

Professor Gordon McVie is a leading international authority in the research and treatment of cancer. He is now Senior Consultant at the European Institute of Oncology in Milan, and Director of Cancer Intelligence, an organisation he founded to improve worldwide cancer outcomes.

Prior to that, as Director General of The Cancer Research Campaign, he joined forces with Sir Paul Nurse of Imperial Cancer Research Fund to combine the two organisations' relevant strengths in a new merged charity, Cancer Research UK, the largest volunteer-supported cancer research organisation in the world.

Is this book any good, and is it any use? Yes to both, so skip the foreword and get on with it! Sharon Morrison writes in a racy, readable style and talks about breast cancer with an authority and insight which the conventional "all you need to know about breast cancer" charity leaflets totally lack.

We've come a long way in my thirty years as a consultant oncologist. Not only medically, but in the realisation that communication about illness is as important to the patient's well being as medical advances.

How I wish I could have persuaded some of my patients in the 70s to read this book. I can't forget the ladies, mostly but not all from the Scottish Highlands, who, on hearing they had cancer, would "put their face to the wall". And, determined to die, they usually did. And frequently unnecessarily, as their cancers were curable. My generation of doctors was taught that the last person to hear the diagnosis was the patient, and only then, if the family gave permission. An early referral to me as the new doc on the block in Glasgow's revered University hospital, the Western Infirmary, was: "Please consider my patient for chemotherapy, but on no account talk about the side effects, and certainly don't tell her the diagnosis." To which, as a self-righteous 31-year old zealot, I replied "get stuffed!" or some such sentiment, dressed up in suitable medspeak. The lady had breast cancer like our authoress but, unlike our heroine in this book, she had had a mastectomy. She heard the diagnosis from me (don't tell me she hadn't worked it out), got chemo, with all the unpleasant side effects, and was cured.

Thankfully we all talk about cancer now: the media, celebs, charities with pink flyers, even Departments of Health. And communication skills have found their way into the medical undergraduate curriculum, and maybe they help patients. So do we need more advice? Given that cancer is the second most searched topic

6

after pornography on the Internet, I think the answer is "Yes".

Nothing can beat the personal account of cancer, delivered in plain English, as this book does. Nothing will better reassure the patient that he or she matters as an individual. Nothing will relieve the nagging uncertainty which the diagnosis brings, but Sharon Morrison does show how to handle it, and how to get on with life in a positive way.

I recommend that newly diagnosed patients read "Even the eyebrows?" and newly qualified doctors, too.

Introduction

As a single parent of three children, working full time, I really don't have time for illness, so when I was diagnosed with breast cancer my first thought was the terrifying-but-normal "I'm going to die." My second was, incomprehensibly, "how long will I have to take off work?"

Once I'd got my head round the fact that I was now one of those cancer statistics, I thought I should take a closer look at them. My findings didn't exactly make me feel great: one in nine* women in the UK will get breast cancer and one in three will have a recurrence. So I headed for the bookshelves to find out more. Well there are truckloads on the subject but, from my own research, they're all pretty earnest, scary and heavy going. Basically for me to recover from cancer and live to a ripe old age, I would need to be an alcohol-free, stress-free, organic vegan who also happens to be an exercise junkie.

When I broke the news to my children they were naturally frightened and upset, but while I had decided to handle the situation with honesty, I wanted to make light of it too, treat it like the massive inconvenience it was. And it helped.

But as "up" as I was determined to be, there were certain reactions that had to be handled very sensitively, for example, my son was horrified when my hair fell out, because he thought friends at school would tease him and make fun of me. I had to help him come to terms with the unavoidable changes in me, and I had to respect his feelings of insecurity. The girls, on the other hand, were more interested in the disease itself and wanted to know why cancer happens and how it spreads. I responded as openly as I could, knowing that there is no satisfactory answer to: "why you mum?"

Once I'd had the tumour removed and started treatment, there were obvious, and some less obvious, changes to my body. I began recounting my new experiences to my children, Merlyn, Jenny and Richard, and we all enjoyed the absurdity of some of the situations I now found myself in. We were all hugely embarrassed too with other predicaments

I encountered as chemotherapy took control of my bowels.

Four years have passed since I was first diagnosed, and the one thing I'm certain of is that attitude is contagious, so it's better all round if you have the right one. When you have a life threatening illness it's a serious business, but I found that by using my imagination to diminish my cancer, rather than build it up and allow it to control me, worked like a dose of, well, Imodium Instants.

Throughout my treatment I worked virtually all the time. I didn't feel on top of the world, but I didn't feel that bad either, yet all you seem to hear of are horror stories about the toll treatments like chemotherapy and radiotherapy take on you. If you have cancer the last thing you need is even more fear piled on you, so here's my response to all those well-meaning scare-mongery books: a guide dedicated to helping parents, children, friends, relatives and employers understand what is happening to someone they love, like or work with, what to expect and how to help. Most importantly though, if you have been diagnosed with cancer, this is dedicated to you.

This is not a long book as you can see. It's not a difficult read either - no navels have been contemplated during its writing nor scientific boffins consulted.

What you see is what you get: a practical account of managing cancer with your boxing gloves on.

*This 'one in nine' statistic is a little misleading. It's actually a lifetime risk, which means one in nine women, or 11% of women in the UK, will get breast cancer during the course of their life. Breast cancer is rare in women under 30, but diagnosis increases with age, so the older you are, the higher the risk. For example, up to the age of 25 you have a one in 15,000 risk of breast cancer, between 40 and 50 that rises to one in 50.

Chapter 1: In denial

꘏

The Pope's not a Catholic, the world's not round, Scrooge wasn't a miser and this definitely wasn't a lump in my breast.

I suspect I would be far from alone in admitting that I have always been a little lax about checking regularly for lumps, despite all the information out there. So it's no surprise that when I did discover the lump in my right breast, it was completely accidental. One night in bed my hand brushed over my breast and I felt something hard. This was not the usual semi-squishy, fibrous stuff I've been familiar with my entire adult life, it felt alien. How strange that such a tiny thing - firstborns excluded - should evoke such mute terror. I kept prodding and pushing it. It didn't hurt when I did this, but it didn't disperse either. So I tried again the following night, and the night after that. Of course I was worried, but I didn't want to tell anyone about my fears, they could be groundless, and I would have made the people I love worry unnecessarily.

I should have made an appointment with my doctor straight away, but that would really mean it was serious, so I decided a Well Woman clinic was the place for me. Quick and anonymous. I made the call, "Excuse me, could I book a mammogram please?" "No problem," came the reply, " why do you want one?" "I think I've got a lump in my breast." "I'm sorry you can't have a mammogram, you'll need to see your doctor." Puzzled, I persevered, "I'd rather have a mammogram. Why can't I do that?" "Because you're not a well woman." Boom, boom.

I am sure there must be excellent reasons why you should only have a mammogram when you think there's absolutely nothing wrong, but I can't for the life of me think what they might be. My advice to any woman who wants a mammogram because she thinks she might have a problem, but doesn't want to see her doctor, is to be economical with the truth. I dithered for another two weeks before making an appointment with mine. A delay of two weeks might have had tragic consequences, yet sometimes you have to wait longer than that to get an appointment with your own GP anyway.

My doctor examined me and uttered a quick "ah" as she felt the lump. I had hoped she'd tell me that it was nothing, instead, but not quite as good, she reassured me that at my age the lump was more likely to be fibrous tissue. I saw the graphs, absorbed the statistics; it all made sense. Fibrous tissue. Good. An appointment with a consultant was made for the following Monday, three days before I was due to fly out on holiday, so I carried on as normal, going to work, getting the suitcases ready, not daring to tell a soul. Was I worried? Yes and no; I kept myself deliriously busy so I had no time to dwell on the situation.

The day of the consultation loomed, but I had to go to London for a meeting first. On the way back to London Liverpool Street station, I popped into Rigby & Peller to be measured for a new bra and try on an amazing swimming costume that, my sister Merlyn informed me, "makes you look 10lbs lighter". I had to have it. Every woman should at some point in her life visit this lingerie store. The assistants know what they're doing, and will help you find just the right size and style. It's a unique experience; wearing one of their bras makes you look better, walk taller, feel fitter but you're a lot poorer, as this kind of underpinning doesn't come cheap. The detour meant I was rushing to make the train, get out of the car park and drive to the hospital. After the hustle and bustle of the last few hours in London, the quiet calm of the waiting room was unnerving. I was keen to get this particular meeting over and done with. The uncertainty felt physically stressful; I just wanted to go home, cuddle my kids, feel normal again.

A nurse showed me into a consulting room where I was introduced to Fiona McNeill, a surgeon specialising in breast cancer. She was confident, reassuringly concerned and very easy to talk to. I felt as relaxed as it's possible to feel, given the circumstances, as she explained what she was going to do to discover more about this lump. She would give me a physical examination, and then conduct a needle test. The needle test would remove some tissue from the lump in the breast for analysis. If the lump was a cyst, the needle would probably pop it and draw out liquid. A mammogram would be taken (at last) and an ultrasound scan made.

I undressed, sat on the bed and Fiona examined me. She felt where the lump was and asked me to lie down while she inserted a small needle into it to extract the tissue or pop the cyst. I prayed for pop. When the needle was removed I could see it contained tissue, not liquid. "Well it's not a cyst, so let's get a mammogram done to see what's there," said Fiona. OK, now I was worried. I was shown into a changing room and given a gown. From there I was taken into a smaller room, asked to stand facing a tall structure with what looked like a griddle pan in the middle. This was the mammogram machine. A nurse flattened my breast and tried to reshape it a few times, before sandwiching it between two metal plates. It was more uncomfortable that I had imagined it would be, but it was over in seconds.

A mammogram is an x-ray of the breast tissue; Fiona would be able to understand more about the nature of my lump from this and discover if there was anything else suspicious there. While the x-ray was being developed, I was shown into yet another room where the ultrasound examination of my breast would take place. The whole process was very thorough, and I knew from everything I had been told by Fiona and had read prior to this appointment, that it was completely normal to do all of these tests if you had a lump.

The last time I'd had a scan was nine years earlier and I saw my son Richard moving around my womb like a slow tadpole and I had felt so elated. This time round, the scan revealed a small, pebble-like shape. My lump. The sonographer (in this case another doctor, who specialised in diagnosing the images transmitted by ultrasound) told me it was about three centimetres wide. As I still only understand imperial measurements, three centimetres didn't seem so bad. While we both stared at the screen, I was aware that Fiona had joined us. If there were nothing to worry about, why would she have bothered to come in? I took this as an altogether bad omen. Good call.

Within only 30 minutes, although it seemed much longer, I was back in Fiona's consulting room, sitting on the edge of my seat. "What happens now?" I asked, trying to sound laid back but clearly looking stricken. "I'm going to send the tissue I took from your breast to the lab for analysis and then we'll talk again." But I'm going on holiday in three days time. "So see you tomorrow evening. Same time alright with you?"

In the seclusion of the hospital car park, behind the security of my steering wheel, I cried. For the first time I felt fear. I might actually have cancer. But with only 24 hours before I'd know for certain one way or the other, there was no point burdening anyone else with this information. In this case a trouble shared would really have meant a trouble multiplied. So I drove home and enjoyed the company of my children perhaps a little bit more than I might normally have done.

The next day was a blur, I was keeping busy in the office but it was hard to concentrate on anything. All

I needed were the test results. If they were negative I could relax, laugh about it and generally get on with my life. I had an evening appointment, but turned up early on the off chance Fiona had a cancellation. She hadn't, so I flicked through countless magazines, not really seeing anything at all, until I was told Fiona was free.

I was so anxious about what she was going to say that I actually didn't hear anything she did say. I knew she was talking to me, but my hearing only began working properly when she said,

"… and we'll need to fix a date for the operation, can you do this week?" Fiona was consulting her diary.

"This week? Operation?" I asked, blinking, as realisation began to dawn.

"It's got to come out Sharon," Fiona replied. I think she guessed I'd missed some vital information.

"I haven't got cancer have I?" It's really odd to hear yourself say those words, and after all the weeks of worrying that I might have cancer, it still had the power to take my breath away.

"Yes, you have cancer," Fiona said.

I stared back blankly, and asked the only question that now mattered, "Am I going to die?"

"Of course not, but we must remove the lump. How does the end of the week sound?"

I am going to die.

This time I didn't wait until I got into the car, I started crying there and then and didn't stop until I was nearly home. Thinking you're going to die when you've been diagnosed with cancer is perfectly normal, de rigueur almost. Of course most of us won't die. Although breast cancer is the most common form of cancer in the UK, with over 40,000 cases being diagnosed annually, death rates have fallen by 21% over the past 10 years. But when that kind of news is delivered, you feel particularly alone, singled out, the only one going through it. It's almost as though no one can feel your particular brand of pain, a little like when you gave birth or lost someone very close to you.

I know I should have fired so many questions at Fiona there and then, but all I did was to take out my diary and agree when the operation should be performed. It would be on the Monday following my return from holiday, just over two weeks from now.

"Surely I shouldn't wait that long, won't the cancer have taken an even greater hold? I need the operation as soon as possible don't I? I'll cancel the holiday."

Fiona smiled and said very gently "There's no point cancelling your holiday, two weeks will make no difference. The cancer's been growing in your body for years."

That comment pulled me up short; it diminished the menace that I felt, made the cancer seem less virulent and within Fiona's control. So the situation wasn't so black after all, just black-ish.

Fiona gave me a small handbook filled with information I would find helpful now that my cancer was confirmed. Most useful of all, not that I appreciated it at the time, was a series of blank pages on which I should write down questions I'd like to ask at my next appointment. As I slowly regained my composure Fiona explained to me what would happen during the operation. The cancer would be removed under general anaesthetic, a small area of tissue surrounding it would also be removed, as would a number of lymph glands in the armpit. These tissues would be analysed to see whether the cancer had spread beyond the breast. The recovery time after this type of surgery is surprisingly quick, so I would only be in hospital for a matter of three or four days.

"Will I look very different?" I asked.

"Not really, you'll lose a quarter of your breast."

I felt relieved, I had thought that she might be talking mastectomy here.

An appointment had already been made with Dr Philip Murray, who would be my oncologist, for the week after the operation. He would discuss my treatment.

"Until we have performed the operation, no one can tell what your treatment will be, but it's most likely going to be chemotherapy followed by radiotherapy and Tamoxifen tablets."

I nodded my head like I was taking it all in. But I wasn't. For the benefit of all of you who may be about to enter into this maelstrom, or if you have friends and relatives about to go through this, here are the questions I suggest you ask, because they are the ones I wished I had at the time:

1. How can you be certain I'm not going to die until you operate?
2. Can you tell whether or not my cancer is primary or secondary from the mammogram?
3. What are the chances the cancer has spread?
4. Have we caught it early?
5. What if I don't want chemotherapy, what other choices do I have?
6. Does size (of the cancer) matter?
7. How many grades of cancer are there and what difference does the grade make to my treatment and recovery?

8. How will my cancer affect the future health of my children, will they now be more susceptible? What about my sisters?
9. What will my breast look like after the operation?
10. If my breasts look different can an operation be performed to make them look the same?
11. One in three women with breast cancer will have a recurrence, where in the body is it likely to occur?
12. What can I do to avoid a recurrence?
13. What's Tamoxifen?
14. What's an oncologist?

Although feeling like I'd been hit on the head with a mallet – and that would have been preferable to having cancer – my sensible side took over. How will this affect my ability to work?

"Sharon, you have a serious illness and the treatment will span a nine-month period. So you should be thinking in terms of taking a few months off. You'll be very tired and you'll need to rest."

A few months off! There was no way I could afford to take a few weeks off, no matter what the experts said. I worked for a small company and had a huge mortgage. Enough said? Worse still, I was about to go on an expensive holiday I couldn't possibly enjoy. I got into the car not really knowing what I should do next, except to go home and have a really stiff drink. Then my eyes fell on the Rigby & Peller bag that, in my distress, I'd left there from the day before. It was carrying the bras and swimming costume, the cost of which equated favourably with the National Debt. Beautiful bras that would only be a perfect fit for the next two weeks. It never rains.

Chapter 2: A healthy outlook

⅋ↄ

I hated school with a passion, so I stayed away a lot. The more I stayed away, the more I hated it. The net result was that I excelled in nothing except manners, an attribute my parents had drummed into my three sisters and me from birth. I was also a natural sloth, so while one sister, Loraine, was a sprinter, the other, Lesley, became captain of the school hockey team and the youngest, Merlyn, went on to play county badminton, I watched television. And I was extremely good at it.

Dad was always encouraging me to go and get some exercise, but I couldn't think of a worse torture. Except for one: sports day. I regarded this highly competitive, annual ritual with such fear and loathing that if I couldn't convince mum I was too sick to go to school on that particular day, I would try to give myself a nosebleed before the races began. I had to do this surreptitiously of course, so banging my nose against the toilet door was my preferred method. Why? I had no agility, I had no speed, I had no technique but most of all I hated losing. I wasn't a bad loser, but I was mortified by failure, so much so I'd rather not participate than run that risk. So, regular as clockwork, more or less as soon as the race had started, I'd fall over. I had no chance of winning anyway, but I hadn't lost because I was the slowest either. It sounds loony now, but it made a lot of sense to me then.

My sisters and I all ate the same meals, but they were all far healthier and slim line. I was your normal miserable fat person who hadn't quite made the connection between my shape and my lack of exercise. I was quite happy to go with the "you're big boned" flow from relatives, less happy to be humiliated by "hey Bessie Bunter" taunts at school.

By some strange twist of fate or the weakness of multiple-choice, I passed my 11 Plus and went to the local grammar school. The competition was so intense I should have thrown a sickey for terms at a time, but mum had sussed me out by then, and there was no choice, I had to go to school. Within a very short space of time I became competitive. No, not because I wanted to "win", I just didn't want the shame of losing again. Someone's got to, but it wasn't going to be me. I spent more time studying and started to improve my grades all the time. I also got to enjoy team sports like rounders and netball, but tennis was obsessive, to the point where, together with three of my best friends, we would play after school in the rain. You could be forgiven for thinking I'd started to turn into a sporting success to rival that of my sisters'. The reverse was true. I remained a hopeless case. If someone could be relied upon to miss a ball, misjudge a shot or generally run the wrong way, it would be me, but I loved the activity. And I started to lose weight. Not huge amounts, but enough to look good (with my clothes on that is) and feel more confident.

Exercise alone is not the key to a healthy and long life. Sadly both my mum and dad, despite their sporty backgrounds, died relatively young from heart disease. Mum was 50 and dad 58. Over the years dad, who had always been a fit man, but on the large side, had become grossly overweight, around 25 stone, thanks to a cartilage injury he'd never had sorted out; mum, on the other hand, was as slim as slim could be, looked under 40 and was still turning heads in the street and cartwheels in the garden. They both smoked though, and that was the problem.

Neither of my parents drank, with the exception of

cream sherry at Christmas, so alcohol wasn't something I was particularly interested in. Straight from college however, I got a job in an advertising agency in Covent Garden and swiftly gained a lifelong interest in it. It was the late 70s, and wine bars with faux Cockney-cool names, like the Brahms & Liszt, were shooting up all over London. They were joined shortly after by a frothy explosion of cocktail bars. 'Happy hours', where you could buy really, really expensive drinks at only really expensive prices, were the norm. This was a time you went out to lunch and had a drink, and then often went out in the evening after work, with clients or with friends, and had some more. The weight started to creep on again, but there were no school friends to play potty games of tennis, rounders or netball with.

As the responsibilities and pressures of work grew, it was increasingly difficult to find the time to do any form of regular exercise, so thank the Lord for Jane Fonda. She revolutionised my life. Her workout video was easy to follow, and helped me keep in reasonable shape. She actually produced the video in 1978, and I still occasionally use it now, 30 years on. She looked great; how was I to know that it took years of intensive ballet training to achieve and maintain a body like that? She was, though, an advocate of healthy eating, probably teetering on obsessively cranky, but it got me thinking about the kind of food I ate, and how I could improve my diet, without being on one. Like most women, I've followed one faddy regime after another, probably for most of my working life, but still wanted to lose weight. The one fact that was clear to me (as well as all the dieticians in the world), dieting really does make you gain weight in the long run.

In my search for the holy grail of weight loss, I discovered food combining, or rather I read an excerpt from a new book by Michel Montignac called *Dine Out And Lose Weight*. Food combining means, as the name suggests, you only eat one type of food group at a time. So breakfast could be a carbohydrate meal, dinner a protein meal. It may sound difficult to grasp, but it's worth sticking with as the upside is that you can eat huge amounts of food, even the fried variety, and lose weight. Why? The enzymes in your digestive system work far more efficiently breaking down one type of food than a mixture. The outcome is that more nutrients are taken from the food and put to work in your body and less laid down as fat. This wasn't new-fangled diet, but one based on a 1930s' regime created by an American doctor to help diabetics. He was called Dr Hay. I wasn't diabetic, but what really appealed to me was that up to one litre of red wine could be consumed a day. Now I wasn't intending to increase my alcohol intake, but this made food combining devastatingly attractive.

To ensure I was getting all the vitamins and minerals I needed, I also started taking supplements, especially antioxidants. The main reason for taking antioxidants was to remove harmful chemicals, also known as free radicals, caused by oxidisation within the body. Free radicals sound quite liberal and friendly, but they're quite nasty, they attack and damage healthy cells which can lead, ultimately, to cancer. As you get older, the natural reserves of antioxidants in the body decrease; the best way to protect yourself from free radicals is, of course, to eat plenty of fresh fruit and vegetables. And I did.

So here I am, a sensible, aware, everything-in-moderation, woman. By 2004 I'd been living a rural existence in a village in Essex for 11 years, in a beautiful tumble down house that I loved. I had three children whom I adored and had breast fed as babies, and was managing director of a public relations consultancy that was, for me, the most rewarding job in the world. As far as I knew, there was no history of cancer in my family, so the chances of me getting the big C, I thought to myself, were pretty slim.

That summer, at my children's school fete, I noticed a young woman taking the dog obedience class, who seemed so familiar, but I couldn't remember why.

"Excuse me but don't I know you?" I asked.

"Hello," she replied, "you're Merlyn's sister aren't you? I'm Claudine. You used to come to my aerobics classes."

We got chatting and I soon found out that this young woman was 45 years old, three years younger than me, but she looked amazing. It wasn't just her figure, but her skin, eyes, her whole demeanour. Without even taking the time to think about it, I asked her if she could become my personal trainer. I've never had a personal trainer in my life but I would be 50 in a couple of years' time and I really did want to look and feel fabulous. Loraine was holding her 50th birthday party in Gibraltar in August, just three months away, another reason to take some action now.

Despite my food-combining regime, I'd adopted a few bad habits: given the choice of a glass of wine after work, or an intensive work out, the wine would always win. I needed some discipline and, as far as exercise was concerned, it could only come from someone else. Claudine and I struck a deal, and started running together three times a week from the following week. After a couple of months I had a newfound energy and I was looking trimmer. I started buying a few summery clothes, skimpier than normal because I knew I could now carry it off. I wasn't looking too bad, with and without my clothes on.

Six weeks before I was due to fly out to Gibraltar, I felt a lump in my right breast. Or had I? The other breast didn't feel the same though. Maybe it is a lump. Each night when I went to bed I would concentrate on making this lump insignificant. I did this for a whole month.

Chapter 3: How do I tell the kids?

🙠

Now my cancer had been confirmed, I would have to tell the children. I was terrified by the thought of it. Instinctively I felt they should know, and Fiona backed this up. As a family we're all very close and I wanted to make sure I handled this news the right way. Honesty, given the ages of my children, was the best policy. As we were flying off to a villa in southern Spain the next morning, the news, like my operation, could wait until the end of the fortnight. We were going from Spain to Gibraltar for Loraine's birthday party, obviously she would have to remain in the dark too. Why spoil her big day?

The first person I told was my sister Merlyn. I waited until the children were asleep then I phoned her from my bedroom. I felt incredibly emotional just dialling her number, and when I tried to tell her I had cancer, I broke down before I could utter the last syllable. As it turned out it was very good practice; every single time I had to tell someone about my illness I would break down. It was clear a fair proportion of people thought whatever I had was terminal. But then, so did I.

Merlyn was upset and wanted to drive over straight away to be with me, but we'd all be on a plane in a matter of hours, so there was no point. We chatted for a while, me keeping my voice down, and agreeing that only her husband Andrew should be told. All our other friends and family could wait until after the holiday.

She asked me many questions, most I couldn't answer, but we were both stricken with the seriousness of what I was facing. Then my bedroom door was flung open and there was Jenny, demanding to know what was wrong. I confess that the wind was temporarily knocked out of me. I had expected to dictate at least when and how I told my children about the cancer and the operation, but here was my ten year old, big blue eyes sparkling with tears, lips pursed tight against her emotion. "I've got to go. Jenny's here," I gabbled down the phone then hung up. Jenny, in her excitement about the holiday, couldn't sleep and had been repacking her case when she overheard my conversation.

I took Jenny in my arms.

"Mum, what's wrong? Why have you got to have an operation?"

Honesty's the best policy, honesty's the best policy, I kept repeating to myself. "I went to see the doctor today because I've got a lump in my breast, and I'm going to have an operation to remove it." I felt far from calm, but thought I sounded it.

"What is this lump Mum? Oh no, it's not cancer is it?"

The realisation and pleading in her voice frightened me, and I found my honesty mantra legging it into the distance.

"It's sort of cancer, well, a bit of cancer, just a little bit, that's why I'm having an operation. It's not serious though, or the doctor wouldn't let me go on holiday would she?"

"But you're not going to die are you mum?"

In her terrified innocence, she had hit home; it was the only thought that occupied my mind. I would die and leave my three fantastic kids without a mum. Now, hearing Jenny's voice, I realised her fear was as great as my own. "No darling, I'm going to live to a ripe old age before I leave you, Richard or Merlyn."

"Who else knows?" Jenny asked.

"Just you and Aunty Merlyn so far, but I will tell Aunty Les when we get to Gibraltar."

I told her that I wasn't planning to tell anyone else until after the holiday, as I didn't want this kind of news to overshadow the birthday celebrations. Now, of course, I would need to tell my daughter Merlyn. Privately I knew my honesty policy should be put on hold as far as Richard was concerned. Judging from Jenny's response to learning about my "little bit" of cancer Richard, my shadow, was likely to react very badly.

Before we knew it, we were on a plane heading for the Costa del Sol and I was going to have a great time. I don't want to make too much of this positive mental attitude thing, but it's always worked for me. My glass has always been half full, never, ever half empty. Having spent my entire adult life working in the advertising and public relations industry I know the importance of projecting the right kind of image at key moments. Acting in a certain way, especially in extreme situations, informs people's opinions, influences how they behave, how they feel. I was now experiencing one of those key moments and I was determined that peace, happiness and confidence would emanate from me. There was nothing remotely worthy about my motives; I believed these positive vibes would rub off on those around me and, in return, make me feel a lot better too. I called it my altruistic circle.

There had been no private moment to tell my daughter Merlyn about my cancer until after we arrived in Spain, and Jenny had agreed to keep quiet because we didn't want Richard to suspect anything. So, the next morning, while Richard was playing with my sister Merlyn's two-year old son, Leo, I went into the bedroom with Jenny to deliver the news. I took a deep breath and said: "Darling, I've got something to tell you and I don't want you to be worried. I've got to have an operation when I return from holiday to remove a lump from my breast." I waited for the news to sink in.

Merlyn looked at me and replied: "OK."

And that was it. OK.

I wasn't sure how to take this non-reaction, I suppose I felt a tiny bit miffed that no emotion had registered on her face, but knowing my daughter, this information hit her hard, but she wasn't going to show it. Over the next few weeks I became accustomed to a surprising array of responses to the news of my cancer. For the moment though, this news was confined to a small number of people. It was strictly need-to-know for now.

My sister had offered to be an alternative sounding

board for my children. If they wanted to know anything at all about my cancer, and I wasn't around to ask, or they just preferred to talk to someone who wasn't their mum, she would be there for them. It was a great idea, one of the most clear-headed and practical steps to take in the circumstances. Children are very robust, caring little adults who, while they are suffering inside, won't want to distress those closest to them. So having their aunt, who was also like their second mum, on hand was incredibly reassuring to them and to me. I couldn't stand the thought that they might be bottling up their emotions because they felt there was no outlet or because they didn't want to hurt me.

Now if you're in the position of being a source of information you really need to know what you're talking about, so a little bit of swotting is enormously useful. Children expect adults to have all the answers, but with cancer it's that much harder to do because there are so many unknowns, but "I don't know" isn't a great response when a child is already in distress. You could get in a book or two on the subject to help but, as I had discovered earlier, they're not always all that helpful or encouraging. I found by far the most useful way of data gathering was by talking to the surgeon, the oncologist and the nurses. This is, of course, with the benefit of hindsight. They will give the most honest answers, providing you ask the right questions. It's up to you how you dress up or soften your answers for your children, but they need to be kept informed; the truth though, even when it's brutal, can be told gently.

Once Merlyn and Jenny had checked with their Aunty Merlyn that I wasn't going to die, the questions they asked were very practical. The important thing here is not just to answer the questions honestly, but also to be reassuring at the same time. Cancer is still regarded with such fear that much needs to be done to dispel the perception of it being a serial killer. And this is the best time to do it as children, like adults, can hoard their emotions until they overflow into unpredictable behaviour. The answers, of course, need to differ according to the age or maturity of the children. But, generally speaking, there's no point in getting scientific, it would just go whoosh! Here's how we handled their questions:

Q. What is cancer?

A. It's what happens when your body starts growing a lump (or lumps) it doesn't need. If the lump isn't removed it can interfere with how your body works, and can make you feel really ill.

Q. Can you catch it?

A. Absolutely not.

Q. How does it spread?

A. If you think of your body like a London Underground map, where the different tube lines are like the blood stream in your body, the cancer cells hop on a tube and travel around the body, and get off wherever they want to.

Q. How long will mum be hospital and who's going to look after us while she's away?

A. The operation is such a simple one; she's only going to be in hospital for a few days, it could be as little as three, or as many as five. I'm going to stay with you for as long as you and your mum want me to.

Q. Will mum be the same after the operation?

A. Of course she will. She's likely to be a bit sore after the operation, so we have to be very gentle with her.

Q. Will mum have to stay in bed for a long time?

A. No, she'll be up straight away, but she may feel a little tired because of the anaesthetic, otherwise you wouldn't even know she'd been in hospital.

It's crystal clear that without the support of my family and friends, at the very outset, I would not have been able to manage looking after the children as well as I did; I don't mean the tangible side of things like the regular meals and bath times, although that does matter. It was more psychological reassurance for them that they were not in any danger of being deserted or overlooked in any way. Their opinions, their thoughts and their feelings mattered. With this aspect of their care more than sorted, I was allowed to concentrate on me and come to terms with the enormity of what I was facing.

The day after I returned from holiday was the day of my operation. I needed to tell Richard what was happening before I left for the hospital, but was dreading the moment. He was the first to come down that morning, so I took the opportunity.

"Rich, mum's got to have a small operation at the hospital today. The doctor found a lump in my breast and it's going to be removed..."

I didn't get any further because Richard started screaming and crying that he didn't want me to leave. He was clinging on so tightly I'd have had to have him surgically removed if I'd needed to leave there and then.

When he'd calmed down a little, but was still sobbing, he asked, "who's going to look after me when you're not here?"

"It's all taken care of," I said. "Aunty Merlyn, Uncle Andrew and Leo are going to stay until I'm fully recovered. That's alright isn't it?"

He dried his eyes, and I could see that he was weighing up the information. He looked at me and his face turned sunny and bright with happiness, "that's brilliant mum!" And off he bounded to find Leo.

Chapter 4: The operation

❧

Private medical insurance isn't something I would ever have considered paying for as I've always enjoyed excellent health. However, throughout my career my employers have included medical cover in the package and, for that, I now felt very relieved. I did not want my operation to be handled by the NHS. It's not that I wouldn't get excellent medical care, of course I would, the same surgeon and oncologist looking after me worked for the NHS too. I just knew I would command more of their time and feel more in control of my own if I was a private patient. As important was the knowledge that I would be in a room of my own, with my own bathroom, it would be spotlessly clean and my family could visit me at my convenience, not the hospital's. There was also a nagging suspicion that, with the NHS, I wouldn't be treated like a grown up and there was the sure-fire certainty I'd be at the mercy of long queues, crowded waiting rooms and lashings of red tape.

So, feeling anything but rested and refreshed after my holiday, I put on my bravest face, kissed my children and told them to come and visit me that afternoon. The operation was scheduled for 11.30 that morning, so we could all have tea together. I turned round one last time to wave goodbye and was suddenly stricken with a fear that almost felt sensational; today was the day when it would be confirmed that my body was wracked with malignant tumours and I'd never see Merlyn, Jenny and Richard again. Of course there was absolutely nothing to suggest I had anything other than breast cancer, caught in the early stages, and here I was, trying to look calm and composed but with my face weirdly contorted as I tried to control my emotions. It was no good. I burst into tears and rushed out to the waiting car, leaving my poor kids staring after me. What was I just saying about grown ups?

Once at the hospital, I was checked in, shown to my room and my sister Merlyn started to unpack the few things I'd bought with me. Fiona, my surgeon, came to visit me and had a reassuring chat about the simplicity of the procedure. I knew the operation was very straightforward and would take no longer than an hour tops. I was going to have a wide excision removal, otherwise known, rather unglamorously in my view, as a lumpectomy. A number of my lymph glands, also known as the axilla, would also be removed from my armpit; now that is glamorous.

As the cancer was near the top of the breast and not too far from the armpit, only one incision would need to be made, so there'd be less scarring. The anaesthetist popped in to meet me and ask a few questions about my general health, and then it was on with the gown and off to the theatre.

As I've never had an operation, I've never been anaesthetised. Well let me tell you, if you haven't already been there, it's fantastic! There is just a moment of the most complete and brilliant euphoria before you fall into a wonderful deep sleep. It seemed like only seconds later I was opening my eyes and Fiona was telling me that the operation had gone very well. The tumour and the surrounding tissue had been removed as well as 19 lymph glands from my armpit. The next stage was to analyse the lot to establish whether or not the cancer had spread.

Back in my room, I felt remarkably well; not drowsy, groggy or sore, but I was aware that I wasn't alone in my bed. A warm plastic bag was nestling by my right hip and when I looked properly, I realized it was filled with blood.

"What's this?" I asked a passing nurse.

"It's only a drain," she replied matter-of-factly, "it collects excess fluid that's forming as a result of your operation. Everyone has a drain after an operation like this; there's nothing to worry about."

I was used to seeing these sorts of bags dripping blood into your body after an operation, not taking it away. For me the most worrying thing was finding out that the drain was actually sewn into my body, vividly reminding me of the character Ugolin in Jean de Florette, who sewed part of his sweetheart's hair ribbon into his chest as a keepsake. Eeyew.

Still, this was a necessary evil as I was now producing something called serous fluid, which was rushing to the site of my wound as part of the body's healing process and there would be too much of it for my body to absorb naturally. Serous fluid is clear in colour, but the blood from my wound was mixed in with it, making the contents look a scary red. During the course of my stay in hospital the drain would need to be changed by a nurse once a day. It wasn't at all cumbersome, just a little tricky when having a shower or going to the loo. For me the simplest solution was to hold the bag between my teeth so it wouldn't pull on my side.

I was told that although I'd probably only be in

hospital for a matter of days, the analysis would take a week. As Fiona was about to go on holiday she said she would rush them through so she could discuss the findings with me personally the following Thursday evening. It was Monday now, so I decided that I would stay in hospital until the results came through. To be brutally honest if discovering you have cancer is the worst thing, the next worst thing is waiting to find out if it has spread. I was lucky in that I only had to get through the next four days, I know that some cancer patients can wait for up to two weeks to find out. As fabulous as it was to be able to watch TV in bed, from the tranquillity of my room, all day long, I just couldn't empty my head enough to stop dreading Thursday and wondering whether I should be "putting my affairs in order". I'm really not a drama queen, far from it, but feeling frightened and anxious was now a full time occupation.

The day after the operation I received my first visit from the physiotherapist. She showed me a series of exercises I should do to keep my right arm and shoulder mobile. The exercises were ridiculously easy, but I was warned not to push myself too hard and cause myself injury. One of the senior cancer nurses visited me and told me that I probably wouldn't be able to go back to work for a couple of weeks, nor would I be able to drive.

I found this shocking, as I felt so good, was I going to feel progressively worse? And why couldn't I drive, was my arm going to seize up? Irrespective of what she said, I would be back to work on the following Monday and I'd be driving there. Maybe I was an actor in a former life, because the show was definitely going to go on as far as I was concerned.

Thursday arrived, but I was told that Fiona wouldn't be able to see me until around seven o'clock that evening. So I kept myself busy with more daytime TV, copies of Hello and OK! and packing. I'd agreed with Merlyn that she should collect me, so the children could prepare for my return. In truth, I wanted Merlyn with me in case the news was bad. I'd been on my own when I was told that I had cancer and I wasn't going to do it again. Not that anyone would allow me to.

My mouth was dry and I was feeling quite shaky as we waited. Moments after Fiona invited us into her consulting room, all three of us were smiling from ear to ear.

"It's good news," Fiona told us. "The cancer hadn't spread, the area around the tumour is clear, as are the lymph nodes."

I never knew relief could feel this great. "So what happens next?" I asked, unable to stop smiling.

"I've already made an appointment with Dr Murray, your oncologist, for next week. He'll outline your treatment, when you start your chemotherapy etc..." Fiona carried on talking, but all I could hear was the word "chemotherapy". Why was I going to have that? If everything was clear, I surely only needed radiotherapy, and perhaps some pills.

"Why have I got to have chemotherapy? There's nothing wrong with me is there?"

I was gobsmacked, but I didn't know why. Chemotherapy is recognised as the best post operative treatment for cancer patients available today. Fiona said I would have radiotherapy, but it would follow the chemotherapy. Apparently the combination of my age (48), the size of my tumour (three centimetres) and the grade (three) meant chemotherapy was unavoidable. Of course I knew that if I didn't want the chemotherapy I could decline it, but I'm not stupid.

As my cancer was oestrogen receptor negative (most breast cancers are driven by the hormone oestrogen, but an examination of my breast cancer cells showed that mine wasn't), I wouldn't be prescribed the drug Tamoxifen (which blocks oestrogen from reaching the breast). Patients who were, could take it for five years, which I interpreted as a further five years of protection. I felt cheated.

Months later my oncologist asked me if I would like my tumour analysed to see if it would be responsive to the new wonder breast cancer drug, Herceptin. Essentially the laboratory would check to see whether my cancer had too many copies of the HER-2 gene. This gene controls how cells grow, divide and repair and too many copies of HER-2 are associated with an increased risk of cancer spreading, but Herceptin (also known as a monoclonal antibody) blocks cancer cell growth and signals the immune system to kill the tumour. It sounded like gobbledygook to me, but good gobbledygook. My tumour tested negative, so I wouldn't need Herceptin. The thing is, my oncologist contacted me and asked me what I'd like to do; I had a choice. At that time the drug wasn't readily available on the NHS, so if you didn't have private health insurance you were either lucky or unlucky. Choice didn't come into it. It's hard to think your life expectancy could have been curtailed because of the lack of a company perk. Now Herceptin has been approved by the National Institute for Clinical Excellence (NICE), so anyone who needs it should, theoretically, get it.

Even though I was dressed and ready to go home, I was still carrying around this rather attractive drain accessory and I asked Fiona if she could cut me lose. It's quite normal for people to leave hospital with the drain in place and change the bags themselves but, as I was going straight back to work, I felt the presence of my drain in meetings could be a little off-putting. It took no more than a few seconds for Fiona to cut the stitch holding the drain tube in place, and I felt much freer with it out.

"What will happen without the drain?" I asked.

"Well your body will still keep producing serous fluid, but that will reduce over time. Depending on the amount, your body will either absorb it or your breast will become swollen with it. If the swelling becomes uncomfortable we can drain the fluid off. All you have to do is give us a call."

I didn't think any more about it. I just wanted to go home.

The children had been busy baking and had put up "welcome home" signs. It felt fantastic to give them all hugs and kisses knowing I was going to be fine; I also knew they needed the absolute endorsement that that truly was the case.

Chapter 5: So what exactly is chemotherapy?

℘ව

Chemo? Keymo? Kimo? I wasn't even sure how to spell it and now I was going to have it. But what is chemotherapy? The word itself has almost mystical powers, conjuring up vivid mental images of frail, shadow-like people curled up on beds, quietly writhing in agony and slowly losing the will to live. In truth I'd never really thought about what it actually was, I just seemed to have this perception of some sort of harsh, evil regime, which had to be endured if you were going to survive. I asked my family and friends what they thought chemotherapy was and, bearing in mind how prevalent cancer is these days, the responses were as varied as they were peculiar. They ranged from "I've never actually been sure what's involved, but I know it's unpleasant" and "it's a large machine you slide into, a bit like the old iron lung machine," (does anyone remember the old iron lung machine?) to "every bit of your body's bombarded by deadly rays" and "it's an injection that lasts for hours."

The best explanation I have is that chemotherapy is a drug (or drugs) that behaves like a guided missile. It is fired into the body to seek out and kill cancerous cells that may have spread from the original site of the cancer to other parts of the body. Cancerous cells are recognised by their ability to divide rapidly, but the trouble with this missile is that it can't differentiate between the normal rapidly dividing cells and the cancerous ones. Therefore your hair, nails, membranes (mouth, throat, stomach, digestive tract) are usually affected too, hence the debilitating side effects. The drugs also lower your immune system's defences by attacking the bone marrow, which means you're also more susceptible to infection.

Because the drugs are so toxic (known as cytotoxic), they are usually administered every three weeks, which gives your body time to become healthy enough to receive the treatment again. There is a whole host of drugs that could be prescribed for you and your cancer doctor (or oncologist) decides which are the right ones for you. He or she will base treatment on the size of cancer, its grade, whether it has spread, your health and age and whether you have medical insurance or you're on the NHS. What I hadn't realised was that you can check the drugs prescribed. Why would you need to do this? Well like most things in life, you can choose the brand leader or go for a cheaper alternative. We would all prefer the best brand as it's bound to be the most effective, but with chemotherapy drugs how would you know if you're getting the best? I called my oncologist and asked for the names of the drugs I'd be on. For the first four sessions I would be given cyclophosphamide and epirubicin and, for the last four, taxotere. One of my friends who is an analyst with a bank, and specialises in pharmaceuticals, looked them up and assured me I was getting the best quality drugs available. If I hadn't been I would have kicked up an enormous fuss - irrespective of whether I was private or NHS. The thing is, on the NHS the cocktail of drugs usually prescribed are less expensive, which means where I was going to have eight sessions of chemotherapy, on the NHS patients might have to undergo an additional four sessions. My oncologist assured me the cheaper versions were every bit as effective as the drugs I was on, but that's not the point is it?

There's a lot of information on the Internet about chemotherapy drugs and their side effects, especially the US websites, but I found talking to others, including breast cancer chat rooms, most useful. Giving the cancer nurses the third degree is also one of the best things you can do. They have in-depth experience of dealing with cancer patients during treatment, and the conversations are generally easier, you don't feel so inhibited about asking the daftest questions. I had an appointment to meet Mary, one of my cancer nurses, at the hospital, so I could start asking those questions that were beginning to stack: How will I feel? How long does each session last? What kind of side effects should I expect? What about my weight? Can I still drink wine? What about driving? Could I be a miracle patient and buck all the trends? Mary was everything you would expect: calm, authoritative, kind and keen to help. Of course all I wanted to know was whether or not I'd lose my hair.

"Sharon, you'll start losing your hair two to three weeks after the first treatment." I asked her whether she was sure about this, and she said that some people didn't lose everything, but on my drugs the hair would go. "Even the eyebrows?" I whimpered.

Mary looked at me and nodded slowly, "Even the eyebrows," she replied.

She then talked me through what happens during chemotherapy and how I might feel, but I kept steering the conversation back to my hair. I've always been a little bit vain, but that's only because I've always felt a little bit ugly. The net result is that I've been wearing makeup since I was 13, so the thought of losing a key feature like my hair, including the eyelashes and eyebrows, was beginning to take on gargantuan proportions. How could I work? How could I face people? How could I go to the shops? What on earth would I look like? There had to be something I could do to prevent this. She told me about the cold cap. If I wore this just before and during each session, it could freeze the hair follicles in my scalp to prevent hair loss.

"Does it work?" I asked, feeling hopeful.

"Sometimes," but she didn't look hopeful.

Mary advised me to talk to other people who had had breast cancer. It would help me to find out first hand what really happens to your body, how you feel both physically and mentally and, most importantly for me, how the treatment would affect your ability to work. I had no savings, no second income, basically like everyone I know, no other means of support apart from my salary and Child Benefit. The mortgage would have to be paid every month and that couldn't happen if I had to survive on statutory sick pay. The stress of having this illness was compounded by the uncertainty of not knowing how I'd keep the roof over our heads if I got really ill.

My trainer Claudine told me about her good friend Mandy who had had a mastectomy and recently completed her course of chemotherapy. So we arranged to meet. My sister Merlyn, my nanny Lucy, our family friend Robert and I sat at the dining table and listened to Mandy as she described how chemotherapy had affected her. She told us a tale of unremitting pain and despair. The constant vomiting after each treatment; the total and complete hair loss; the peripheral neuropathy (that's pins and needles in your hands and feet to you and me); the two stone weight loss (there is a God); the arthritis, the dental problems; the bone-deep fatigue; her inability to work throughout the whole period and the fact that she now felt unable to return to her salaried job.

Our eyes were fixed on her throughout; we were stunned, horrified, depressed. Every negative about the treatment had been confirmed. I was going to suffer and there was no way out of it. Mandy only then mentioned that she had a rare blood disorder which meant her reaction to the drugs prescribed was unusually severe. Ah.

Through Mary I was introduced to Helen. Like me she had a grade three cancer, and had been prescribed similar treatment. Unlike me, tests showed that her cancer was oestrogen receptor positive, which meant she could take the anti-cancer drug, Tamoxifen, for five years. Her approach to dealing with the treatment made me feel relieved. She'd got it, she'd dealt with it, and it didn't get in the way of living. That's just how I felt I should treat the treatment too, but it's always helpful to be able to chat to someone who's been through it, especially if they don't have a rare blood disorder.

Helen and I met up for lunch a couple of weeks before my chemotherapy was due to start and she had brought some photos with her. Now I could see the different stages of baldness in living colour, talk unguardedly about other side effects and generally soak up her experiences. I didn't like everything I heard, but I also realised that you could take chemotherapy in your stride. Helen had.

As you will be well aware, medical insurance cover has many benefits. For me it meant choice. Amazingly I could have chemotherapy administered in a private room at the hospital or I could have it at home thanks to a wonderful organisation called Healthcare at Home. Home treatment is available on the NHS too but only in certain circumstances, if the patient is too ill or unable to leave his or her home, for example. Otherwise you would be one of several patients having the treatment at the same time and in the same room. For some this is a real help as you can chat about the changes to your body, exchange views and even have a laugh with fellow sufferers. For others who'd prefer more privacy, just don't want to talk, or don't feel "up" enough for company, this is torture. I opted for home treatment. I'd feel more comfortable and, more importantly, my children could see chemotherapy in action. As could my sisters. Merlyn was with me for every session, and Loraine and Lesley flew over from Gibraltar to be with me whenever they could. It's common sense I know, but understanding dissipates fear and I believe that being able to watch me having cups of tea, chatting to my wonderful nurse Elaine, and generally being relaxed during each session was an enormous relief to everyone. Me too.

The day arrived for my first chemotherapy session, but I had no time to be apprehensive, as I had to attend a client meeting that morning. (I had been told to have a very peaceful day before the treatment to prepare my body for the drugs, but circumstances at work made this impossible.) The meeting ran on and I had to race home to be there before Elaine. We arrived virtually at the same time, and then a procedure began that would be replicated over the next six months. I would sit in a comfortable chair with a drip next to me, a hot wheat bag, straight from my microwave, placed on my arm to warm it up before the drugs (which had been refrigerated) were administered. While I was being warmed up, Elaine would ask me all sorts of questions before showing me the drugs and confirming the dosages with me. She would then insert a cannula into my hand, through which all the chemotherapy drugs would be injected. First though, a saline drip was set up, this would dilute the drugs as they were injected into my veins; a necessary precaution as chemotherapy drugs are, literally, poisonous and would seriously damage my veins without dilution. As it is, the drugs damage the veins anyway, so you generally have to change over arms for future treatments when one becomes too painful for intravenous medication. I had to keep changing arms after my fourth treatment.

In addition to the chemotherapy drugs, anti-sickness medication and steroids were also injected, so the whole process would take between two and three hours. The first session passed off without incident, and the children were home from school in time to see me "plumbed in". Once Elaine had left, the children and my sister Merlyn kept checking that I was still OK. I actually felt no different, but nevertheless we all waited for me to spontaneously combust.

Chapter 6: The hard man haircut's not me
ജ

I always wanted great hair, the sort of hair that people would gossip about, or just admire from afar. I wanted a style that never moved no matter what gale force was blowing, and had great shape and texture, a real Sharon Osborne creation. I wanted boyfriends to ask girlfriends why they didn't have hair like mine, and husbands to argue with wives that they should spend more time on their hair.

When your hair looks good, you feel good too. Sadly my hair's always had a natural kink to it, so unfashionable today, but even with some help from my daughter's GHDs, I tended towards a slightly untidy, out of control style. Now that my hair was falling out fast, I never loved those wayward locks more. If I could have stuck them back in with glue I would've done it.

I'd never had to consider what it would be like without hair, but now I started to feel sorry for all those men I'd ever berated for comb-overs.

The nurses, surgeon and oncologist would talk to me about "when your hair starts to fall out", but I just wanted to know how it falls out. Would I wake up one day like Samson and it's all gone? Or would this be a more gradual process where the hair gets a little thinner over time till there's none left? Elaine said it was best not to towel dry my hair or rub too hard, if I was to stand the greatest chance of keeping it for longer. They all said I'd keep finding more and more of my hair on my pillow in the mornings as time went on, and I might want to consider a very short haircut as the hair loss is more manageable. I can remember how it was when my children were babies and I'd find these beautiful delicate hairs decorating the cot blanket. Perhaps it would be like that.

You know the old adage: if you fail to plan, you plan to fail? Well I knew in my bones I'd never lose my hair, but on the off chance these experienced practitioners might be right, I needed to be prepared.

If I wanted to carry on as normally as possible, I'd need to look as normal as possible. I wasn't prepared to try the bald look (blessed with Grace Kelly features, I might have thought otherwise) so I'd need a wig. My sister made a call to my hairdresser Antoinette Beenders, who immediately went to her favourite wig shop and picked out some styles she thought would suit me. The shop was called TrendCo in London, and I made an appointment to try on these wigs. Merlyn came with me, not just for moral support, but also to prevent me from coming out looking like Hayley Cropper from Coronation Street or even Dolly Parton. Don't get me wrong, their wigs suit their personalities but they do look like wigs. If I was going to have to wear one for the best part of a year, I didn't just want something to cover my head; I wanted a total head makeover.

Once inside this wig emporium I was in awe, there was shelf upon shelf of fabulous looking hair. "Wig" almost seems a derogatory term. These were works of art, and I decided to try them all on, and in every colour. And I did. This is not a process that should be rushed either as wigs are not cheap. (We're talking around £80.00 for starters, and you might need two of them, but shops will deduct the VAT if you're undergoing chemotherapy. You can, in certain circumstances, get wigs free through the NHS.) So I took my time and listened to the invaluable advice of the assistant. The process was very enlightening, as I came to realise that every conceivable hairstyle I had ever liked, but had always thought wouldn't suit me, didn't. Now I knew for absolute certain that a sleek Jennifer Aniston cut was out of the question for me. I kept narrowing the choices down and eventually went for a shortish, chunky cut with plenty of highlights and height. She was called Roni. The assistant cut the wig a little while I was wearing it so that it framed my face better. I have to admit, even without makeup and in my worst comfy gear, I looked OK. Two hours at TrendCo beat clothes shopping any day.

Now to show my kids. They would be kind, they would be critical and best of all they would be truthful. My sister gave me a polystyrene head to keep the wig on, and that's how I showed my new hair off.

"Come on mum, try it on so we can see," they pleaded.

But I said "not yet" as we'd organised Sunday lunch at a new restaurant, and I was going to give it a test drive then. When Sunday finally arrived I was unbelievably nervous. What if the wig looks awful? What if the kids hate it? What if a hungry seagull takes a fancy to it and plucks it from my head? What if a spark from someone's cigarette makes my completely manmade creation burn to a frazzle while still on my head? All perfectly natural fears, and ones that made me, superwoman, feel disturbingly vulnerable. I got dressed quickly, so I could spend more time preening, and then made my grand entrance downstairs. Only my sister had seen the wig in situ, so to speak, so her husband Andrew and my three kids were sort of looking forward to the event. There were plenty of "Ah, it looks lovely", and "you wouldn't know it wasn't yours" and "really suits you." So I felt far more confident when we entered the restaurant. The lunch passed off without any seagull or cigarette incidents and, when I paid the obligatory visit to the loo for more preening, I looked at my perfect hair, patted it and exited.

So I was organised when, exactly 19 days after my first chemotherapy session, the "will it/won't it?" suspense was over.

I was at a meeting with a new client on the Friday morning (the 19th day) and that afternoon was due to drive to London with the children for my sister Merlyn's birthday party on the Saturday evening. I'd arranged to have my chemotherapy three weeks prior to the party, as I was told that you'd be feeling your best just before the next chemotherapy session. Making a simple decision like deciding on the timing of treatment was good for me. It made me feel far more in control of my situation. Once you've been diagnosed with cancer, you can feel a little incidental to the procedures you have to undergo, so it's good to do things that remind you that you are number one. Anyway, back to the meeting.

It was a rather long one, but every time I moved my head, I was aware of seeing some of my hair slowly floating down onto my shoulders. When I say "some" that really doesn't describe the disconcertingly large amounts that were beginning to fall out. By keeping my head very, very still I managed to stop the fallout temporarily and, at the end of the meeting, walked very carefully back to the car. The area behind the driver's seat resembled the floor of a hairdressing salon; my shoulders now had fur epaulettes. It had started.

When I got home I had a practice shake of my head. Bad idea. I tied a very large scarf around my head, turban style, got the vacuum cleaner out, started cleaning the car and then worked my way through the house. I had to face facts; I was moulting.

That scarf remained in place during the journey to London and throughout the night. I presented myself to a hairdresser in Canary Wharf the next morning and asked her to shave my head. This all sounds very matter of fact doesn't it? Well it wasn't. I was mortified and upset. I had really thought I'd keep every last hair on my head. So when I was standing in front of the hairdresser I was actually trying to ask her to shave my head, but I couldn't get the words out, so I broke down instead. She was a wonderful, gentle Geordie, who had obviously dealt with many women like me. She asked a few questions and told me, "I'm not going to shave your head, it will be too much of a shock for you and your children. I'll cut it really short now, so everyone can get used to it first."

The more she cut off, the more I cried. I'd had short hair in the past, but as short as this style was going to be, there would be no style at all within the next few weeks. I felt ugly and unfeminine. All my family and friends coming to the party knew I had just started chemotherapy but none, with the exception of my sisters, my children and Andrew, knew about my hair loss. Although Roni and I had had a dry run a few weeks earlier, the party in the afternoon was going to be the real acid test.

At my sister's I showered, put my face on and got dressed. I glanced at Roni on her own polystyrene head and took a deep breath. I put her on, played around with her a little and was very pleasantly surprised. I actually looked better wearing a wig than I did with my own hair. I joined the party, accepted all the compliments on how well I looked, and experienced a real high afterwards when I learned that not one guest knew I wasn't, well, quite myself. Now for work.

I work with a great group of lively and supportive people. They all knew I'd bought a wig before I started my treatment, but didn't know I'd be wearing it on the

Monday. Again I felt a little nervous but told myself to get over it. So I did. No one knew (or at least they didn't let on) that I was wearing a wig, and one of the girls thought my hairdresser Antoinette had restyled my hair. When I got home that night, despite having a shorter-than-short Annie Lennox cut, the hair loss was never ending and I couldn't stand it. Lucy brought in her mum's electric hair clippers and my children, Merlyn and I all took turns to shave my head. I looked like Uncle Fester from the Addams Family after a diet. If I felt unfeminine before, it just got a little bit worse.

A couple of days later I was buying my lunch at the local Spar, when one of the assistants noticed my new hair.

"You've got a new hairdo! Looks nice."

I thanked her and was about to leave when another assistant came up. She scrutinised my hair and I began to feel a little uncomfortable. She knew. Was she going to rip it off and announce to the rest of the customers that I was actually cheating, and I'd bought nice hair?

"I bet you got that in London," she was nodding at me knowingly.

"Kensington Church Street actually," I replied edging towards the exit.

"Well it looks fantastic," she added looking very satisfied with her judgement.

I told myself that I must stop feeling so self-conscious, but this hair admiration thing was so unusual for me. My wig was everything I thought it would be and, after a few days, even I forgot I was wearing one. Buoyed up with even more confidence I felt ready to face London and clients.

During the normal course of events I would be in London for meetings two or three times a week. That meant a 60-minute train journey from Colchester to London Liverpool Street Station, followed by a walk, tube or taxi ride. On this occasion I had a meeting at Spitalfields, so it would only involve a short walk. I got to the station early for a change, I usually cut it so fine, I have to race everywhere, but I had made up my mind I was going to take things a little easier from now on. I waited on the platform, every now and then catching the reflection of my perfect hair on the glass covered hoardings.

The PA system suddenly sprang to life and announced that a fast train was coming through and we should all stand well back from the edge of the platform. The roar of the Norwich to London express was getting louder and louder, and before I could utter "toupée glue" a most violent and cruel wind began circling my head. Its long sinewy fingers were picking at the outer edges of my wig, doing everything it could to dislodge and then throw my pride and joy into the path of the train. I had visions of Roni blowing past all these commuters on platform three who would pretend not to notice and me standing there completely bald but acting oh-so-nonchalant. There was no place for calm here, only blind panic. I had to act fast. I snatched my mobile phone from my bag, clamped it to my ear, and held on to the hair closest to the phone with my thumb and forefinger, with my other hand, I pressed my fingers over the ear, ostensibly to hear better, but securing the other side of the wig at the same time. The intercity train rocketed past in a noisy buffeting blur, and I shut my eyes and held on tight. It worked, but I knew my mobile phone was now a vital part of my outdoor uniform.

When my train arrived, I got on, noticed some admiring glances, this time from men, and sat down quite pleased with myself. When I eventually took a sneaky look at my reflection in the train window I was horrified. All the hair on the top of my head was now ramrod straight and bolt upright; I couldn't have achieved a better effect with a wet finger and an electrical socket! When I thought no one was looking, I gently patted my hair back down again. What else could go wrong?

With each passing day, my scalp was becoming

increasingly itchy, so much so, that I began to feel ill just looking into my wig before putting it on in the mornings. On my way home from work, I would whip it off as soon as I got in the car throwing it onto the passenger seat. My sleek, even-shaped head was now decorated with teenage lumps, bumps and pustules. I sought advice from nurses, doctors and wig wearers, who examined my eruptions with a great deal of zeal. All had conflicting comments. It varied from the mystifying: "ah, you've not been moisturising have you?" to the reasonable: "you've got a fungal infection in your hair follicles. You can get treatment for that," to the inconceivable: "you've developed an allergy to the wig." What a choice. I could look good and feel sick, or I could just look gruesome.

I've never, ever worn any kind of headgear, not even when skiing, I just look terrible, and I have witnesses who would readily testify to this, so the thought that I'd have to come over all ethnic and go around wearing scarves filled me with dread. I also remembered seeing pictures of Princess Caroline of Monaco, Princess Grace's daughter, (I have a thing about that family, don't I?) years earlier, looking drop dead gorgeous in a headscarf. She was suffering from alopecia at the time. Without drastic plastic surgery I could not carry off the scarf thing. I had to find a solution fast.

I decided on some self-help and started wearing a barrier between the wig and my scalp. This barrier took the form of a sewn up stocking top - the sort bank robbers wore over their faces pre CCTV - and actually came supplied with the wig. The stocking was to secure and control your own hair under the wig. As I had no hair, I hadn't seen the need to use it. But I did, and the reaction was as dramatic as it was soothing. The spots disappeared overnight.

Wearing a wig has been very necessary, not just for me but for my children. There would be times when I would have to visit their schools or we'd go out somewhere together and looking "normal" was important to us all. For my son Richard the wig became a crucial component of our lives. At home I wouldn't wear my wig, and Richard became used to visitors looking a little shocked when they met the new me. So he started closing the curtains or running at me with my wig if he thought anyone might see me through the windows. His concern wasn't selfish but protective. He didn't want anyone to make fun of me. Equally I understood that, inevitably, some children might poke fun at him. So, while I wasn't about to start behaving differently at home, I wasn't going to put my children through any additional pressure about my appearance outside it, they'd had enough to cope with already.

The great thing about kids - and I'm talking about quite a broad age range from eight to fourteen years - is that they're very accepting, understanding and generous. Both Merlyn and Jenny would invite their friends to the house for tea, having briefed them about me beforehand, and they didn't bat an eyelid between them, although they were obviously curious. Soon Richard started bringing his friends home too and the boys, like the girls, behaved as if nothing had changed. Gradually Richard came to feel easier about my public appearances (as did I).

The biggest test for both of us came when I decided to treat the children, Robert and Lucy to a weekend break at Center Parcs in Suffolk. I'd actually planned this a few months earlier and thought I'd have more hair than I did when the time came. My hair had started to grow back after my fourth treatment, so I now had a steel grey coating of very short hair, but as the hair had started growing back, my eyebrows, eyelashes, fingernails and toenails decided to do a disappearing act. Nevertheless, I decided that I wouldn't take my wig, this was going to be an activity holiday, and I couldn't think of anything worse than sitting by the side of the pool, because I was wearing a wig. I was going to participate.

To make the holiday special, I'd booked us into a

show where a buffet dinner was part of the deal. We did the queuing for food bit and took our places to be entertained. The quality of the show was so poor, it was actually hysterically funny. All the kids, not just mine, loved it. Then the serenading began. The lead singer, in a truly terrible wig and matching outfit, and his spotlight, were slowly making their way across the dance floor. To Jenny's horror the spotlight fell on her. She looked up into the eyes of this 40-something crooner who held his hand outstretched to her. Of course she was meant to gracefully take his hand, and dance with him in front of hundreds of people. She'd just turned 11, so whatever he had planned just wasn't going to happen; she quickly pushed his arm away, which meant he was twisted towards me. The spotlight followed him. The same hand was now outstretched to me. I would have given anything to be in a different place and I was also conscious that my new hair must, in this bright, bright light, look like a silver halo on an egg. To have spurned him a second time though would have been hugely embarrassing, so I did take his hand, and I did dance with him in front of those hundreds of people and I enjoyed the applause at the end.

When I returned to my seat, Richard leaned over, patted my arm and in a very serious voice pronounced, "Mum, you were very brave, I'm very proud of you."

And I was proud of him, because I can only imagine how he must have felt seeing my hard man haircut and me on such public display.

Photographs

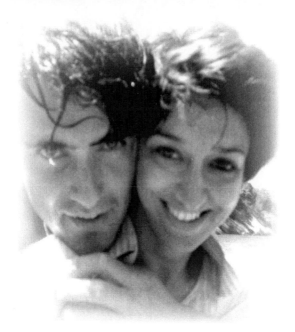

On holiday with John in Crete.

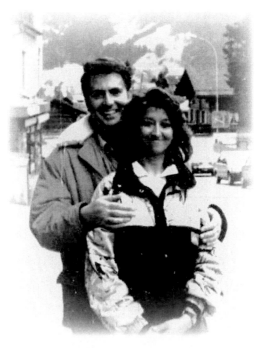

Skiing in Chateau D'Oeux, Switzerland.

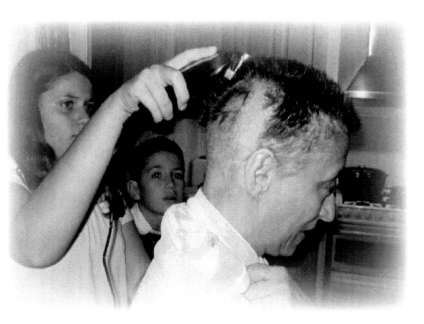

Jenny and Richard bravely lend a hand to shave my head.

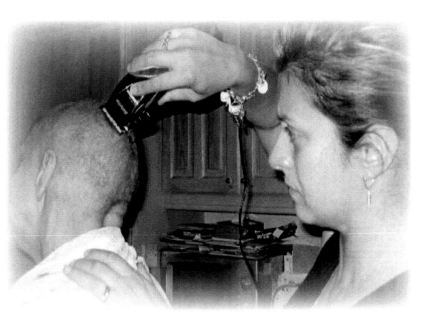

My sister, Merlyn, finishes the restyle!

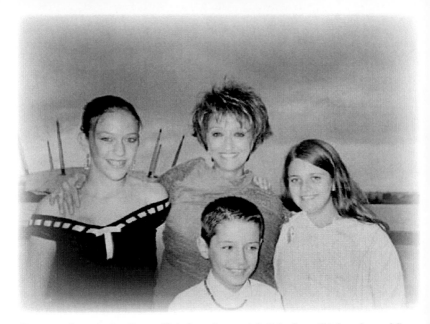

Giving the wig its first official outing with Merlyn, Richard, and Jenny by my side.

Nick, Leanne, and the girls, Victoria, Katherine, and Elizabeth.

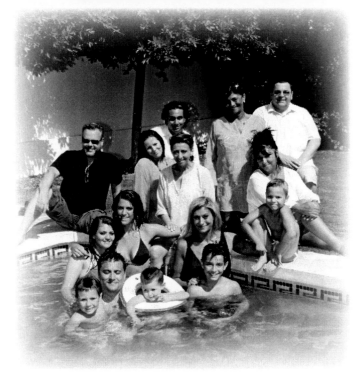

Relaxing by the pool in Spain.

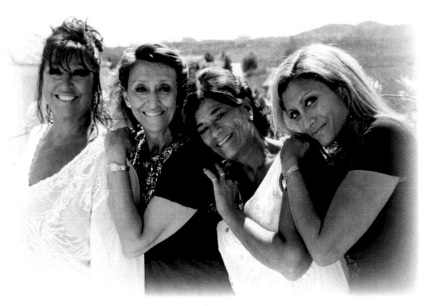

Precious time together for Lesley, me, Loraine and Merlyn.

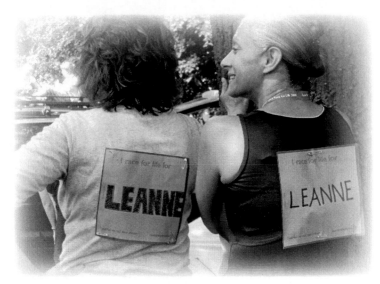

Completing Race for Life with my sister, Meryln.

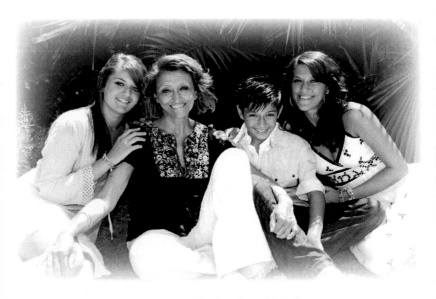

Jenny, me, Richard and Merlyn.
Back to normal – hair, eyebrows, everything.

Chapter 7: Shit happens

ℰℋ

There's an awful amount of information on diet when it comes to post operative care. You're advised to go organic, to drink specific veggie shakes to bolster your immune system, to cut down on this or cut out that. There's also plenty of advice on how to dress and do your make up when you're bereft of hair. And let's not forget the menopause, the onset of which is triggered by chemotherapy; well there's more on that subject than you could ever read. But what is missing is frightening. It's frightening because you don't know you need the information until it's too late. By which time you could have died of embarrassment, not cancer.

The kind of situations I'm talking about are truly awkward and sensitive, yet the crucial help and practical guidance on dealing with such incidents just don't exist

– if they do, I haven't found them. Now I'd coped very well with hair loss, but then everyone knows that you're probably going to lose your hair, so I made sure I had the wig as my fallback position. These are all very obvious subjects to tackle, but what about the less palatable areas? What about the diarrhoea? Although every book and website has noted that this particular affliction *could* be a side effect of chemotherapy drugs, no one goes on to deal with the next steps. For example: do you sit on the loo for days on end just to be safe, or can you go to work and carry on as normal, safe in the knowledge that your body will give you ample warning to find a toilet?

I can now tell you from my own bitter and personal experience that you don't need to sit on a loo for days on end just to be safe, but you will wish you had. One week after my third chemotherapy session, I was attending a meeting in London. I had just left the building, when I felt the most extraordinary sensation in my stomach and bowels. It was as if all my organs had decided to vacate my body incredibly fast. Sadly what was vacating wasn't organs, just weeks and weeks' worth of food and by products. Crap in other words. So there I was, in the middle of London, frozen in time, wondering how I was going to move the next few inches, let alone get to my train station. It was a crisp December afternoon but I was hot and sweaty with panic. I needed to find somewhere to get cleaned up, but I was terrified of moving in case my knickers and tights couldn't contain the nasty deposit I'd involuntarily made. I started to picture this smart businesswoman - me, briefcase in hand, with a truly terrific hairstyle, leaving a trail of excrement behind, like a human snail. This image was as horrific as it was real. I saw the sign for a public loo and headed for it. I wanted to run, but I had to waddle, taking the tiniest of steps to ensure my load stayed put. Once there, I disposed of everything in a carrier bag I had with me (thank heavens for small mercies), then ventured out, bought some wet wipes and returned to the loo. My intention was to get really clean before getting on the train home in time to see Jenny and Richard in their school's Christmas play. Today of all days I just couldn't be late, I chided myself, but then that organs-vacating-now feeling came over me once again, and I had no choice but to sit there. After a while, I realised that if I didn't make a move I'd never be back in time for the play. It was now or never. I made it to the platform and boarded the train. The feeling of panic had not left me, and I desperately wanted to head back to the sanctuary of the toilet as I was already envisaging the dreadful scenario that could unfold during the hour's journey on that train. So I purposefully sat myself right next to the toilet, on the aisle seat, and as soon as the train moved out of the station, I would bolt in there and stay put. It seemed the most logical thing to do. I'd feel much safer and I'm sure the other passengers would have agreed with me had they known.

The train set off, and before it was even out of the station, the loo door next to me slammed shut. A young lady had gone in, and didn't exit until the train stopped at Colchester, my stop too, a gut-wrenchingly, buttock-clenchingly 60 minutes of misery later. How I made it through that journey I still don't know. I folded my arms around my stomach, bowed my head and concentrated on commanding my bowels to behave themselves. If ever I needed to demonstrate that the mind could control bodily functions, it was now. And I did it.

I later confided in my sister Merlyn who, practical as ever, put together my emergency shit kit: scented nappy sacks, night-time sanitary towels, wet wipes, spare pair of knickers and Imodium Instants. And from now on, I never, ever left home without them. I had many close shaves throughout my treatment, but at least I was prepared. I felt I had learned an unnecessarily harsh lesson, but I shouldn't have been in that position in the first place. I needed to be given more advice and information, but at least you know now. When my treatment was completed I thought my bowels would settle down into a normal routine once again. They haven't and I dearly want predictability back.

One of the other side effects I suffered came completely from left field. It wasn't covered by any of the notes that accompanied the chemotherapy drugs, which at least diarrhoea was. So you could have knocked me down with a feather when my fingernails and toenails just started flaking off. This happened after my fifth chemotherapy session. It was a nuisance, as I couldn't even put a jumper on without one of the nails catching and causing me some toe-curling moments. Worse than that was the ugliness of it all. My fingers now looked quite unsightly, so much so when we had presentations to make at work to our clients, I would get one of my colleagues to press the buttons, show the boards and generally do everything to ensure I didn't have my hands on display. As my feet weren't on show, I only had the pressure of shoe leather on nail-less toes to contend with. Painful, but not unsightly.

It's sometimes hard to put your finger on what exactly was the worst side effect of the treatment. Certainly the diarrhoea attacks come top of my list, whereas I always thought it would be hair loss, which actually comes second. Losing my sense of taste also hit me hard. I love a glass of wine or three and, at a testing time like this, it would have been a small reward to relax with a crisp chenin blanc, but I was resigned to drinking sweet white wine and apple juice, as anything else tasted awful. Even a strong cup of tea first thing in the morning was disgusting. And the same went for food too. I just didn't know what I wanted to eat. Sweet things definitely had the edge, as did nursery food like fish fingers and jacket potatoes filled with baked beans. When I then developed mouth and throat ulcers, which sometimes made it hard to speak clearly or swallow painlessly, my life was complete.

You would think the absence of taste and the presence of ulcers would at least help to keep your weight at bay wouldn't you? No such silver lining. Although I continued to watch what I ate and to exercise moderately three times a week, none of it could prevent me from gaining a few pounds. My oncologist told me it had nothing to do with the treatment; I was just putting more food into my body than it was burning off. I actually believe the onset of the menopause is nearer the mark.

Add to that insomnia - a common affliction for cancer patients, but not one I had been told about - and I felt truly grotty. I would have looked it too if it weren't for the miracle of camouflage makeup and that darned fine hair.

As I described earlier in Chapter Four, the exercises prescribed by the physiotherapist for me, were rather too easy. Well they were until a few days after my return home. With each day that passed just stretching my right arm out became increasingly painful. I was concerned that if I kept doing the exercises, I might be doing myself more harm than good. I also noticed a strange bony line forming under my right armpit and running down my arm to my hand. This didn't seem right, so I called the hospital and arranged a physiotherapy session, as I assumed I'd just been doing my exercises incorrectly. The physiotherapist was cheerful and clearly in rude health. After filling in all the usual forms, she asked me to lie down and slowly raise my arm. As I did this, I began to feel the familiar pain.

"Ah there it is," she said reassuringly. "You need to be pinged off."

Pardon?

"The lymphatic vessel in your arm has become hard and is pulling, a bit like a taut string. It's called cording."

It was a new one on me. "It could disappear on its own, but that might take some time. So we could ping it off now."

"Does it hurt?" I asked. I'm not a wimp, but she was already manoeuvring herself into a position above my head, with a very strong grip on my wrist and elbow. What ever she was about to do to me, it would be without the aid of anaesthetic.

"Try to relax," she called from somewhere in the distance. Then she pulled my elbow up towards my head with all her might. That really hurt. "OK. I'm going to try again," she said as she took a deep breath.

"Oh God," is all I thought.

She grasped my elbow and arm, lifted up slightly and pulled again. And I felt a ping. It was a brilliant ping, because all the tightness and pain just disappeared. She assured me that I was unlikely to get any more cording, but showed me, my sister Merlyn and my daughter Jenny how to ping off unwanted lymphatic vessels.

It wasn't long, a mere 24 hours in fact, before pinging off was necessary again. My sister wasn't there, so I asked Jenny to do it. I lay down on the living room floor as Jenny tried her best to 'break the cord', but to no avail; I did manage to do a couple of circuits of the living room floor, on my back, without getting carpet burns though. And all the while my elder daughter Merlyn was looking on in disgust, telling us how gross we looked.

As with most things in life it pays to be given slightly more coaching than we were, so Jenny and I went back for another session (or lesson) with the physiotherapist. She was surprised to see us, but showed us what to do again. Luckily, Fiona, my surgeon happened to be there and called in to see me.

"Ah, you've got cording."

At least I now realised it was quite common, it's just that absolutely no one had mentioned it to me until I asked. Fiona then told me that as I had had quite a lot of serous fluid forming, I was likely to have more cording. I'll come on to the serous fluid bit in a moment, but I wanted to let you know, that for the next few weeks, I was able to ping off on my own before I went to bed, so relieving Jenny of quite a horrible chore and Merlyn the embarrassment of watching it.

You may remember that Fiona had told me my right breast could become swollen with serous fluid as I'd had the drain removed early. Well that did happen, but I hadn't realised how much it would ache the bigger it got, or that it would reach and then surpass Jordan's proportions (pre her breast reduction), which it very quickly did. And it went on for weeks. On three occasions I actually thought my breast would explode; it was that gargantuan, I had to go to hospital where the fluid was drained off with a syringe. At business meetings I had to wear tops that draped rather than clung, as I looked so lopsided, but for me it was still better than having to carry that drain accessory around with me. And I know I was fortunate to still have most of my breast. After a couple of weeks the swelling subsided, but I'm still lopsided as my Jordan boob is now small and pert, shame about the other one.

Exactly one month after completing chemotherapy I started radiotherapy. The idea of blasting the site of the tumour with powerful x-rays is to completely cleanse the area. I wondered why this was needed, as chemotherapy appeared to be so ruthless in attacking everything, but my oncologist assured me that it was a necessary, but far less evil, partner to chemotherapy.

The treatment would last for 20 days, which meant a month of Mondays to Fridays visiting the local hospital and waiting my turn. The information given to you from the hospital was very straightforward and led me to believe there was nothing to worry about. I asked as many people as I could how they felt about radiotherapy and their comments ranged from "you'll feel really sore," and "it makes you so tired you just want to go to sleep all the time," to "it's a walk in the park."

I don't know why, but for me the thought of radiotherapy held no fears; it sounded gentle, non aggressive and fast. In practice, I discovered it was all those things. But then after chemotherapy, with all that it entailed, how could a little bit of zapping be intimidating? And the speed of the procedure - just a matter of minutes from start to finish - meant I had my treatment on the way in to work each morning. My right breast did eventually get very sore and was sunburned in appearance, and I did peel, but that was the sum total of my discomfort.

In fact my only frustration was in trying to find a parking space at the hospital that had a fantastically small car park. Although specific appointments are always made for each out patient, many decided to arrive extraordinarily early to get a parking space. For someone like me who tends to cut things fine, it meant I ended up parking streets away and had to race to get to my appointment in time. By now, I looked on this minor inconvenience as an opportunity to get some exercise and fresh air.

Chapter 8: When the going gets tough...

꿍

I have saved this chapter till near the end because it is so fundamental to how you handle the whole kit and caboodle. If you're rich and famous, independently wealthy or don't have to work to keep the roof over your head, you probably don't need to read on. Unless you're an employer too of course, then please stick with it, because you need to know how your support - or lack of it - can deeply affect your employee and his/her long-term health.

We all know employers can be ageist, sexist or chauvinistic, basically all the ists, but never more so than when it comes to protecting their business. And nothing gets them going quite like "I'm pregnant" and "maternity leave". Throughout my working life I've lost count of the number of times I've seen raised eyebrows and looks of utter despair when an employer finds out his or her employee is pregnant. Of course, not all employers are like this, but recent research commissioned by the Equal Opportunities Commission found that up to 30,000 pregnant women are illegally sacked or forced out of their job every year. It's appalling, but at least becoming pregnant is usually a choice or a happy surprise, and the systems are in place to ensure your rights, as far as work is concerned, are protected. Getting cancer is obviously not a choice, and the surprise is definitely a nasty one.

When I was pregnant, with each of my three children, I carried on working up to the day I gave birth. This wasn't because I was forced to, but because I didn't feel unwell or incapable of handling my job. In fact I believe working kept my mind off the downsides of pregnancy (ditto when I worked throughout my cancer treatment), so I never suffered with morning sickness, cravings or fatigue, quite the opposite in fact, I seemed to have boundless energy. On the other hand, I knew quite a few of my friends soldiered on at work feeling terrible, but not wanting to give their employers any cause for complaint, while others couldn't wait to take maternity leave because they felt that was the only way they could enjoy their pregnancy.

When undergoing treatment for cancer it's virtually

impossible to calculate how much time you'll need to take off work; you don't know how you're going to react either physically or mentally. And, what if you have to take six months off, who's going to pay you? Sure, there's statutory sick pay but the amount is so small could you pay the mortgage, let alone all the other weekly and monthly bills on it? Not a chance. So you have to rely on your boss to do the decent thing and look after you.

"Looking after you" can take a number of different forms. Having job security, and therefore money, is crucial, because not only does this knowledge free you from stress at an incredibly stressful time, it means you feel mentally more robust to cope with the treatment and its side effects.

If you're a senior member of a large successful company, the chances are that you will get as much time off as you need on full pay. I know of three large organisations (and I'm including a local authority in this) that have actually continued to pay key personnel their full salary for six months in one case, 12 months in another and an amazing two years in another. If you're a junior member of the same company, you are unlikely to be so lucky. If you're in a small company with dwindling profits, or one that's encountering tough trading conditions, chances are your boss can't afford to be so generous financially. But he or she could find a way to keep you motivated and loyal, while getting some work out of you when you're having your good weeks. This requires a degree of thinking outside the box, as well as a few drops of humanity.

Well I am a senior member of a small company, which, at the time that my cancer was diagnosed, wasn't in the best of health either. My chairman, who also owned the company, took a very hard line with me. From the moment I returned to work after the operation I was badgered at every opportunity. He even called me at home on the two days I took off for chemotherapy and, on one occasion, was shouting so loudly at me, my sister could hear him from the receiver. I felt too weak, and quite shocked, to fight back. But there was more to come. Just before we broke for Christmas my boss said he needed to meet me to discuss some business issues before he went to his holiday home in France. Could I make the 28th December? I naturally agreed and suggested my house as the venue.

The gist of the meeting was to basically inform me that I had not been performing, drastic steps would have to be taken to remedy the situation and I was in the firing line. Scary stuff, but sadly that wasn't all; two weeks earlier my ex-husband John, my partner of 24 years, the only true love of my life and the father of my children, had died very suddenly. I was half way through my chemotherapy by then. I was completely devastated, my children were in shock so, treatment aside, I couldn't have been at a lower ebb, nor felt more vulnerable than I did when my boss visited me at home.

I defended myself as robustly as I could that day, but all the while I just couldn't believe anyone would apply this degree of pressure on someone who not only had a serious illness, but was also suffering from a dreadful personal loss. My boss obviously felt he was doing the right thing, and it forced me to consider my options, all of which seemed bleak. I looked at protecting my mortgage payments through insurance, but having cancer excludes you as a candidate. I thought about getting another job, but that's hard when you don't have hair and nails, plus you'd have to ask for time off for treatment; hardly a great employment prospect. But the fear of losing my job, when it was virtually impossible to find another means of living, given my circumstances, literally made my brain freeze. I found it difficult to have any rational thoughts whatsoever. I couldn't see white for the black; I couldn't feel safe for the chasms of uncertainty, but most of all I was headlights-in-the-eyes terrified.

I had not told a soul about my business pressures,

although everyone was aware I was working rather too hard at a time when I should have been taking it far easier. I decided to confide in my sister Merlyn and told her the predicament I was in, how low I was feeling, and that I wanted help. That was all I needed to do: ask for help. And I got it within 48 hours. Now I had a solicitor (pro bono thank goodness), telling me exactly what my rights were, and what my next steps should be.

Then Merlyn started to tell a few of our very close friends and, before I knew it, I had an army of supporters not just rallying round and making me feel more confident, but giving me the very best business advice on handling my current situation with my boss. I felt buoyed up by the immense support they were giving me and I could almost see their arms locking around me to protect me.

The worst aspect of all of this is that I had worked hard for the same company for seven years, becoming managing director after four. We'd been through thick and thin together, but all of a sudden I was definitely on the way out. Can cancer really be so threatening? Well clearly it can, and I found myself in a pitch battle for my livelihood, when I should have been concentrating on fighting for my life.

But what if you don't have family and friends who

can rally round, or access to top-flight legal help? My advice, and this is based on particularly bitter experience, is to stand up for yourself. There's plenty of information on your employment rights that you can get from the Citizen's Advice Bureau and your local library, or you could just call the editor of a reputable Human Resources magazine, like People Management, and ask for their recommendation on the best website to interrogate. You may not feel very brave or confident, but you have done nothing wrong, and cannot be forced to go. It's very strange, but I found the very act of making a stand, despite being petrified, made me feel more in control of my situation and far stronger. Don't forget too, the last thing an employer wants is the cost of a court case and the negative publicity that goes with it. Trust me, I'm in PR.

I am still working at the same agency and for the same boss, I am still the managing director and I am still passionate about my work. My boss rates me and respects me, but we still argue about his treatment of me. I truly believe my cancer frightened him and made him think only about the short term. In a country where more and more women are in full time employment, and one in nine women (remember this is a lifetime risk) will get breast cancer, employers will be dealing with this incredibly serious illness on a more and more regular basis. So they have to wake up and smell the coffee. It's not rocket science, but staff who are treated with respect during what is for them an intensely traumatic period, will return to work more committed, loyal and positive. Everyone's a winner.

Chapter 9: Going hippy

D id you know that 50% of people undergoing chemotherapy don't need it? It's a stop-you-in-your-tracks kind of thought when you're about to start your course of chemotherapy, as I was. Yet I'd heard it straight from the horse's mouth, well the Steve Wright show on Radio Two. Steve Wright was interviewing an American doctor (I assumed he was a doctor, I tuned in too late to know for certain) who believed that chemotherapy drugs shouldn't be automatically prescribed to treat cancer as there were plenty of other treatments. By the end of the interview I had I dismissed this view as that of a sad old tree-hugging evangelist.

A couple of days after hearing this programme I met a friend of my sister's whose relative had recently been diagnosed with cancer. I mentioned the date when I was due to start chemotherapy and she asked me, with a slightly critical-quizzical look on her face, "So you're going ahead with it then?" Up to that point I didn't think I had a choice, but this arched-eyebrow question, coupled with the comments from the radio interview, now made me feel ever so slightly ill-informed, stuck-in-the-mud and sorry for the tree hugger. I lamely asked, "What's the alternative?" Well "alternative" is a key word as I then found from Google. There's a confusing array of treatments based on strict dietary regimes, light therapy, dendritic cell therapy, heat shock protein therapy, mega doses of vitamin C and so on. The list is a long one but, frankly, I got bored.

Some sounded a little sensible while others were verging on the insane. What was worse, to my mind, were the false hopes these alternative therapies would undoubtedly raise in people who were at their most vulnerable and suggestible. In my heart of hearts I knew that the only route I'd take would be the one backed by decades of robust research and clinical trials with a graph that demonstrated an exponential success rate. And that was clearly and unequivocally chemotherapy; who was I to argue with that kind of evidence? I'm all for upsetting the applecart and being a little anarchic when necessary, but now was not the time to take uncalculated risks. Give me the science any day.

Reading about the alternatives was invaluable in another way because I learned about complementary therapies. These are treatments that work alongside chemotherapy to help your body cope with the side effects of the drugs and generally make you feel better. These complementary therapies essentially break down into two areas – psychological and physical, and incorporate the following disciplines:

Psychological	Physical
Counselling	Massage
Meditation	Aromatherapy
Hypnotherapy	Acupuncture
Art therapy	Reflexology
Self-help groups	Shiatsu

Any of these can be used throughout the term of your chemotherapy, as long as it helps to make you feel great at a time when you know you are going to feel rubbish. The psychological (or mental) approach is invaluable if you find dealing with the reality of cancer a steep hill to climb. You need to be able to discuss or express your feelings, if not with family and friends, then with professional therapists. Only by getting your head straight can you feel more positive about your situation, avoid depression and handle the three-weekly kick in the stomach more stoically. I never felt down or horrified at the thought of my treatment, for me the worst was over; the cancer had been removed, I was going to live and the chemotherapy was a very necessary evil, so self-help groups or counselling would have been wasted on me. Besides, I talked about my cancer and treatment openly and easily from the outset and had many kind souls whose only intention in life, it seemed to me at the time, was to listen, sympathise and support. Not everyone would find themselves with such a network of minders, so I count myself lucky.

No surprise then that I was immediately drawn to the physical therapies, essentially those that could, in different circumstances, be regarded as pampering. Who wouldn't want a regular massage, especially with aromatherapy oils? Not a single parent of three children, working full time, that's for sure. I would even add manicures, pedicures and visits to the hairdresser to the list too, obviously not an experience worth having for me as I eventually lost toenails, fingernails and hair. But the thought of an hour's pampering, with no special occasion in sight, sounded like heaven. I had heard from one of my chemotherapy nurses - way in advance of having the treatment - that one of her patients, Helen, had had reflexology during chemotherapy and found it very helpful. I knew vaguely that reflexology was based on Ancient Egyptian, Indian and Chinese foot massage techniques and that each part of the foot corresponds to specific organs, glands, bones and muscles. So, by applying pressure to one part of the foot, pain or symptoms could be relieved in another part of the body. Reflexology could also restore and maintain the body's natural equilibrium. When I met Helen for lunch to discuss her treatment and experiences in more detail, she told me she believed her positive physical response to treatment was improved thanks to reflexology.

Frankly the thought of someone playing with my feet and toes for an hour meant more to me than maintaining natural equilibrium ever could; I just had to check it out. And that's when I encountered my first problem. I rang a couple of reflexologists in my area, but they refused to treat me because I was going to have chemotherapy! They, and I can now include some health and beauty spas and salons in this too, believe the act of massage would counteract the benefits of the chemotherapy, or in the worst case, cause the cancer to spread through the circulatory and lymphatic systems. I was appalled and angered by this. How could a chemotherapy nurse, dealing with cancer patients every single day, recommend this, and a reflexologist or masseur contradict it? My oncologist would know what to do. Thank heaven for the voice of reason.

"If you think reflexology will make you feel better during the treatment, then you should have it. It won't harm you, and it won't affect the efficacy of the drugs one iota," said Dr Murray with a resigned look. He's obviously been here before.

"Do you think it will help me through the chemo though? Is it worth doing?" I asked, even though I'd now made up my mind to do it, just to spite the opposition.

"If you want to do it, you should do it."

"But will it improve my chances?" I pleaded.

"As far as I'm concerned you're cured," he replied. "The chemotherapy's just to make absolutely sure." He obviously doesn't rate reflexology.

I finally found Jenny Holben, thanks to my osteopath Simon Bacon. I met her and we chatted about what the chemotherapy drugs were going to do to my system and how this form of treatment could help. Jenny told me the most important thing was to ensure my immune system was constantly tuned up, because of the battering it was going to take. She also wanted to help me recover properly on my right side, the shoulder and breast specifically. So, one week before my first ever chemotherapy session, Jenny came to my home and gave me my first ever reflexology session. She was very gentle and explained where I was, well, out of tune I suppose, and what she was going to do to counteract this. After an hour, which was perfect bliss by the way, I was left thirsty and tired. Thirsty because this therapy, like massage, helps to eliminate toxins and is therefore also dehydrating; tired, because it was so completely relaxing.

These treatments were hugely beneficial to me. I enjoyed them, looked forward to them even, and didn't really suffer too badly with the side effects of chemotherapy. I also got a whole new vocabulary. Now I was talking about meridians (energy zones to you) and chakras (we've got seven) like they were going out of style. I think I must have gone hippy! But now my treatment is over, I've continued with my reflexology sessions, one a month, because I'm worth it.

How much of my great reaction to the effects of chemotherapy is down to reflexology is hard to quantify, because I used other "therapies" too. Jenny told me that it was very important to get plenty of fresh air in my system to aid my immune system whilst it was being attacked by the drugs. I'm not exactly allergic to fresh air, and I think the air conditioning in my car must help, but walking when I could take the car has seemed very odd to me for some time. Longevity was now very important to me, so I did something about it. Three mornings a week, at six o'clock, my trainer Claudine and I would fast walk two and a quarter miles around the village. This gave me fresh air and exercise. Now the treatment's over we're jogging 15 miles a week – an amazing feat for a sloth like me. I've been told that jogging's a dreadful exercise that jars the bones, and hurts the joints, and I agree, I think jogging stinks, but I get a real sense of satisfaction when I've completed the circuits. And I'm fitter and healthier; if I can have a bottom like Cameron Diaz through doing this, I think I might just carry on.

To really boost my feeling of well being I wanted to get a good night's sleep, but I'd become an insomniac almost from the start of my chemotherapy. I should have been exhausted, having the treatment, working full time and looking after the children and the house. Actually I was exhausted because I just couldn't sleep. So I felt (and must have looked) like a zombie, 24/7. When I mentioned my plight to Elaine, my chemotherapy nurse, a couple of sessions in, she said that steroids usually have this effect and I could have sleeping pills if I liked. Yes please, anything that could make me drift off at night and stop thinking; anything that could me look fresh and alert rather than grey and haggard. Bring it on. Elaine brought diazepam, also known as Valium. Part of the benzodiazepine family, it comes from a long line of successful sleep inducers, but taken long term it can become addictive. Still, I needed to sleep, so I took one an hour before bedtime and looked forward to a great night's sleep. I waited and I waited, but it didn't happen. The next day I asked Elaine whether I needed something stronger; she checked with my oncologist, and suggested I take two, rather than one. That night and two diazepams later, I was still wide-awake. The next night I tried my own prescription: two diazepams with loads of wine - I was desperate for sleep after all. Still no good. I then asked if my oncologist could prescribe Zopiclone. This is a non-benzodiazepine; I had used it once before when I wasn't sleeping well, and it had worked. Strangely my doctor had told me it was non-addictive, so I assumed that it wouldn't have been as powerful as Valium in counteracting the affects of the steroids. Well, it was. From the moment I had Zopiclone, I slept like a baby. I even looked forward to going to bed, because I would drift off to a fantastic night's sleep and wake up feeling refreshed and alert. Now I understand you're only supposed to take these pills for about a fortnight or so, but I took them for almost eight months and it was great.

All good things must come to an end, so when my

course of radiotherapy was completed, Dr Murray said I must start weaning myself off Zoplicone. I decided I should forget the weaning bit and just stop. I had had so many different chemicals in my body, not to mention the x-rays, I really thought enough was enough. The net result of my resolve meant I became an insomniac again. For a couple of weeks I was averaging one or two hours' sleep a night, and I was back to looking and feeling dreadful.

Claudine to the rescue: "Have you thought of listening to ocean noises to calm you down at night?"

Er, no. "Quite frankly Claudine, I'll try anything," I replied. I was sceptical as I couldn't believe any kind of music or relaxation technique would work, but you never know. Claudine dropped off a CD, which I played that night. I was instructed by a very boring and monotonous voice to start relaxing every part of my body, and then the wave noises started. I have to confess they did sound nice, but 30 minutes later I heard my CD player clunk off. This was very disappointing, as I don't think I should have been awake to witness that. I persevered, but in general, I had reverted to my average of one to two hours' sleep again.

Over the months, my sleep pattern is improving, and I am generally getting a full four hours of continuous   sleep a night. Which may not sound like a lot to you, but it's a real achievement for me. I am working on building this up to five or six hours if I can.

Now this working mother of three, constantly buzzing with adrenalin, has calm on call. I feel healthier, full of peaceful energy and more in control of my life than I have ever been.

Chapter 10: Half way there

I'd come to the end of my treatment, had check ups with my surgeon and oncologist and all the signs were good. Sadly I'd put on around fourteen pounds in weight, despite regular exercise, and my knees and feet sometimes throbbed as though I'd climbed K2 in flip-flops. I was officially in remission; quite when remission ends I don't know, but I felt lucky to be here, aches and pains and all. The fact that I had come through everything as well as I had was a bonus. I wanted to celebrate in some way, mark the end of an awful period and the dawning of new and exciting phase in my life. With my 50th birthday approaching, I had the ideal opportunity.

The first thing I did was to ask for help. Pre cancer I had always relied on me, it wasn't that I couldn't rely on others, I just didn't want to put busy people under more pressure. Now I felt fine to ask, because I knew my family and friends wanted to be more involved. Merlyn would take care of invitations, follow ups and numbers, Robert catering and accommodation, my sisters and children would help prepare the house for the big day. All I had to do was draw up the guest list. Teamwork's great. I benefit from it every day in business, why I hadn't thought of using it in my private life before now I'll never know.

The last birthday I celebrated with a party was my 30th; I would have celebrated my 40th too, except that I was heavily pregnant with Richard. Now I wanted everyone who had been so worried about me to see that I was in good health; more than anything I wanted to renew acquaintances that I had long ago allowed to lapse. Between work and my weekend job as children's chauffeur, I never found the time, but it's a very poor excuse and I wanted to make up for it now and let everyone know how much I appreciated their support. I had been genuinely touched to know there were so many people rooting for me when they learned about my cancer, and I felt it helped on an emotional level too.

Being realistic, I knew that some people might want to buy me a present, being sensible I knew I should tell them what I wanted: a portrait by Natasha Kerr. I'd come across Natasha's work at an exhibition and fell in love with her style. Her portraits are more a pictorial summary, a visual collage of memories. I wanted to create an heirloom for my children, something they could keep and then pass on to their own children. Getting cancer showed me how fleeting life can be, and if I was going to die before I felt ready, I'd really like there to be a record of my passions, my loves, my life.

Everyone contributed toward the cost of the portrait and it was unveiled, yes I actually cut the ribbon, at my party. It's not every day you reach half a century, and it was all the more shocking because I still felt 23, but it was a great day that became a great evening and then a great morning after the night before.

I had invited Nick, my financial adviser, and his family to the party. He and his wife Leanne have three young children under six. I was especially looking forward to meeting Leanne because she had been diagnosed with breast cancer shortly after my diagnosis. Like me she carried on working, looking after her children and running the household while undergoing chemotherapy and radiotherapy; unlike me she had a mastectomy. She looked beautiful, energetic and vigorous. She was following an exercise regime too, and had already lost two and a half stone. We admired each other's curly hair and it was hard to think just a few months earlier we were both completely hairless, pumped full of drugs and masquerading triumphantly in wig and full make up.

About three weeks after the party, I received an email from Nick that made my heart sink. Leanne had secondary breast cancer in her spine. I called him straight away to find out more. Apparently Leanne had had some pain in her knees and back and went to get it checked out, a bone scan showed there was something on her spine, the MRI scan that followed confirmed that it was cancer. To have come so far, and then to learn you've got to go on that difficult journey again, is devastating. I knew that secondary breast cancer was, more likely than not, terminal. Later I spoke to Leanne. She was calm, composed and chatty, "No we haven't told the children yet, but we will, we want to be as honest as we can. I've spoken to the specialist and I'm told I've got between five and seven years. Bugger!"

My sentiments precisely. There was nothing for it, I spent that night in tears. I was crying for Leanne, crying for Nick, crying for their three children but, guiltily, crying for me too. We've all cried when we've heard about sad situations, but to me this was so personal, so painful, and so real. For the very first time all I could think about was the unfairness of it all.

Shit happens, as I mentioned in an earlier chapter, and you have to deal with it the best way you can. I came across a poem by Michael Josephson, What Will Matter, which made me think about how I might deal with life now:

> "...*what will matter is not what you bought but what you built, not what you got but what you gave*
> *what will matter is not your success but your significance*
> *what will matter is not what you learned but what you taught*
> *what will matter is every act of integrity, compassion, courage or sacrifice that enriched, empowered or encouraged others to emulate your example...*"

I could go on, but you get the drift. If you get cancer, you have two choices: you either get on with life, or you don't. I'm getting on with life because there are so many things I want to do. I'm not talking Kilimanjaro, white water rafting or good works here, but silly little things: one is to wear false eyelashes - don't ask - the other is to jump into the deep end of a swimming pool. For as long as I can remember I've always been too frightened to jump into the deep end, yet I've been swimming all my life. Jenny, my reflexologist, came up with a possible answer to this: "maybe you're frightened of getting in over your head." Me, the female equivalent of Lancelot? I'm frightened by lots of things like half a dozen thugs running after me with baseball bats screaming "let's get her", the supernatural, eating offal, but getting in over my head? What a weird thought.

The morning after talking to Nick and Leanne, I hit the phones. I wasn't going to hang around, I needed to know where I stood, so I wanted to have every scan, x-ray and blood test available on the market, and preferably right now. My knees, which were always painful, had become even more painful, my neck and shoulders felt sore, probably because I'd been spending too much time at the computer, but this was no ordinary soreness, it was obviously cancer again. This time I shared my fears with my sisters and my friends. My oncologist and surgeon both told me that scans were unnecessary, but if it made me feel better then I should have them. I did and they were clear.

So should I get my affairs in order? No, apart from making my will. Should I embark on serious good works of some nature? I'm sure I should but I have a mortgage to pay after all. I have resolved to carry on carrying on; I will continue to embarrass my children in front of their friends, lust after Ralph Lauren furniture, become depressed about the size ten jeans I will never,

ever squeeze into, and look forward to the summer. More specifically I shall look forward to the two weeks every August when the whole family chills together by a pool somewhere and plays endless games of Black Aggie and Scrabble. That's what my life is about and I like it just the way it is.

I might though, when no one's around, jump into the deep end of the swimming pool and see what happens. I'll remove the eyelashes first.

Post Script

When you have cancer you know that those dearest to you are going to feel a lot of pain. As much as you try to minimise it, you can't stop it. Throughout my treatment I did my best to behave as normally as possible. It wasn't always easy, but I felt routine would be a natural comfort blanket at a very uncomfortable time in all our lives.

Once it was all over, which for me was around ten months after the chemotherapy and radiotherapy courses had been completed, and I had a luxuriant head of short, bouncy, wayward curls, I asked those I lived and worked with, as well as my oncologist and reflexologist, to give me a written snapshot of how my cancer affected them. Their stories, as brief as they are, are as important as my own.

Richard, eight years old
⁊꙲

I was upset when I found out mum had cancer and had to have an operation. She was never sick, never. I knew cancer was dangerous and I just didn't know if she was going to live or die. When she went to hospital to have the cancer taken away I didn't know if she was going to come back. I missed her so badly when she went away. It felt like the family had broken up. When I went to see her in the hospital I was so happy. There was a machine that made delicious hot chocolate.

When mum left hospital she had to start having chemotherapy. She had this on Tuesdays at home, so when I got back from school she'd be sitting in her armchair with all these tubes running into her arms. I didn't know that mum would need chemotherapy after the operation, and I didn't know what that meant either.

I think she was about halfway through her treatment when I realised that the tubes contained drugs that would make her better. She enjoyed being with us in the afternoon, having tea and cake together and talking about this and that. She'd usually be at work, so we never got to do these things very often.

I didn't tell my friends at school about mum's cancer, although I could tell the teachers knew something. I wanted to keep it quiet because I didn't want to talk about it. I told my best friend, Connor, who lived around the corner but went to a different school, and he'd keep checking how mum was and was always trying to cheer me up. Connor was the only person I could trust to keep my secret.

Mum told me she was going to lose all her hair, and she bought this wig so she could still carry on going to work and looking normal. Even though she'd worn the wig to a restaurant to try it out and she'd tried to prepare me for the time when she would be bald, I didn't have a clue what it would really be like. One night mum was taking a long time to come up my bedroom to say goodnight, so I went onto the landing to find her. She was looking at her hair in the mirror and crying. She didn't see me though, and I went back to bed. I knew that she must be quite worried about losing her hair.

When it happened I hated it. Mum's wig was brilliant and I wanted her to wear it all the time, even in the house. I felt so embarrassed when people came to the door and she didn't have her wig on because you could see they were a little shocked, even though they tried to hide it. I felt protective of mum but uncomfortable too. I wanted to feel normal but couldn't. I didn't like mum going out anywhere, except to work because then she would definitely wear her wig.

Then dad died and we were all so sad. Mum wore a furry hat to the funeral and then everyone came back to our house. She asked me if she could take her hat off because her head was getting hot, but there were too many people and I didn't want anyone to laugh at her, so I said no. Later, when there weren't so many people about, I went up and told her she could take her hat off, so she did.

When mum's treatment had finished she treated all of us to a trip to Center Parcs. I was very nervous because she told me she wasn't going to wear her wig although I begged her to. She stood out a lot because her hair was so short, I mean really short.

I feel a bit stupid that I was so sensitive about mum's hair when there were more important things to worry about, but what can I say, I was eight?

Jenny, ten years old

I found out mum had cancer by accident. I didn't mean to listen at her bedroom door that night but she was crying and mum wouldn't cry unless it was something serious, so I was worried. She told me she had a lump in her breast and was going to have a small operation to remove it, but it could wait until after our summer holiday in Spain and Gibraltar, and that I mustn't worry. I felt better because you wouldn't go on holiday if you were really sick would you? Mum lied to me, but I was glad because it meant I could enjoy the holiday. I got a little upset when we were in Gibraltar because one evening mum was standing by the quayside watching how fast Richard could run, and I started to realise that the lump in her breast must mean she had breast cancer and you die from that. I asked her if she had breast cancer and she

126

said she did, I asked her if she was going to die and she said she wasn't, but I felt nervous.

When mum started her treatment I thought she managed really well. Even if she was feeling awful, she always looked and acted as though everything was ok. I didn't know what chemo was, but it didn't seem so bad. We'd get home from school and she'd be sitting there with a drip in one arm and a cup of tea in the other, chatting to her nurse, Elaine. Then she'd love to sit by the fire and watch old episodes of Friends with us and laugh her head off. I thought mum needed to look forward to something, and watching Friends in the evenings was it. The house was usually full of people dropping in to lend a hand when needed, but we had our quiet times too. I think mum liked it that way. I did.

In preparation for her hair loss, mum had her hair cut short, then very short. So it helped me adjust to the moment when she had none. I helped shave her head when there was so much hair falling out it was becoming a nuisance.

Mum definitely looked good with the wig on, but I didn't care whether or not she wore it. When my friends came to the house they had been briefed by me beforehand so knew what to expect; sometimes their younger sisters, who didn't know mum was bald, turned up too, so we all got used to some fairly big eyes, open mouths and white faces.

At first I didn't tell anyone about mum's cancer, but someone from school came to a lesson to talk about cancer, so I thought this was my cue to say something. All my friends were very concerned, they comforted me and told me everything was going to be fine. My friends and my teacher would always ask after mum and my teacher wanted to make sure everything was alright at home, not too stressful and whether I was able to do the homework. I said everything was fine, because it was. Thinking back I should have said it was too stressful and got out of the homework.

I wish I could have removed all the money worries so mum didn't have to keep going back to work. She wasn't sleeping at night, and then she'd work all day and sometimes she looked so tired. I told Aunty Raine that I was going to write some stories and make some money, but I didn't get very far with them.

We tried to make the weekends as relaxing as possible for mum. I'd tidy her bedroom, put some magazines out, and order her to go to bed. After a couple of hours Merlyn, Richard and I would bring up a cup of tea and lie on the bed with her chatting.

Throughout everything we all behaved normally, as though chemotherapy was normal, not sleeping was normal, wearing a wig was normal, and being bald was normal. Being normal meant we all coped really well. I feel good about that.

Merlyn, sister

I can best describe Sharon as my sister, mother and best friend rolled onto one. I am the youngest of four sisters; Sha is the second eldest with a nine-year gap between us. Mummy died when I was just nine years old and Sha quite naturally became my mother figure. As I grew up Sharon was working in London at Ogilvy & Mather, I saw her life as exciting and glamorous. She taught me so much about who I wanted to be and what I wanted from life. When I left college I lived with Sharon and John, I was at the birth of their first baby as she was at the birth of mine. As adults we have shared a lot but on the whole up to this point Sharon had always been my rock.

Sharon's phone call came late, the night before she and the kids were flying out for our family holiday in

Spain. Sharon's voice was quiet and calm and controlled at first but full of pain. Her words felt like they were stabbing me in the heart and truly rocked me to the core, but I automatically went into carer mode. We both cried as silently as we could, I put the phone down and collapsed into Andrew's arms. In a way it made the fact that Sharon was on her own even more poignant, I hated the thought that she had faced all of this anguish for the last few weeks by herself. We have shared so much happiness and heartache, but she had not been able to share this fear with me, I couldn't take the pain away; I felt helpless. Like mother, like daughter. Sharon lives her life like our Mummy, never wanting to burden any one, always protecting her family to the nth degree. I was determined that she would not have to face anything else on her own. It was my turn to look after her.

I knew nothing about cancer, chemotherapy or radiotherapy; I had so many questions, I needed to know more. One thing I was certain about was that if Sharon's consultant felt it was necessary, we would not have been going on holiday, she would be on that operating table. Of course, her main fear was for her children and I was able to reassure her that Andrew and I would always be there for them, in every way, so I hopefully was able to comfort her on that score.

I am so very proud of Sharon, she has been so dignified in her recovery. As a family we have always triumphed over adversity, but this was a test of such magnitude and Sharon's tenacity was admirable in the face of the tumour, treatment, awful side effects and John's death.

I was stunned at the treatment Sharon received at work. She had been so totally dedicated to her company and had thrown herself into her work with even greater intensity when she was diagnosed, instead of slowing down. If the truth were known, I took more time off for Sha's chemo sessions than she did. I was constantly on her case as she was supposed to rest the day before a session but, more often than not, her nurse Elaine and I would be waiting for her to dash back from work for her chemo. Her boss showed absolutely no gratitude, his lack of compassion was never more obvious than after John's death when he "put the boot in". I cannot stress how important it is that employers understand that, when everything is so uncertain, the need for job and income stability is essential for a full recovery.

For most people this would have been the final straw, but thankfully Sharon finally shared her troubles with Andrew and me. I put my foot down. She had been Superwoman dealing with all the hardship, determined that she would keep things as normal as possible for the children, so it was hard for me to watch her crumble, not because of the cancer, not because of the loss of her life long partner, but because of her boss who should have been supporting her. Still, in the face of all of this she was loyal and did not want to let her team down. I had to force her to come to the doctor and I argued with her in front of him to take his advice and take time off work and still she wanted to reduce the time he was suggesting. She took four weeks off, and used that time to grieve for John and be with her children.

If ever I had prayed for a lottery win it was now, I just wanted her to be able to stop! Stop worrying about money, stop worrying about work and look after herself for a change. I feel very sad that when I read this book that there were times when Sharon could not ask for my help; I so wanted her to lean on me and allow me to look after her. I have been at every meeting with her consultant and oncologist since.

When she was diagnosed we looked for books that would help us, but not one gave us a practical insight into what we should expect and what we should do. This one does.

Yvette, work colleague

❧

The first inkling we had at work that Sharon might be ill, was, ironically, from a client who knew her sister Merlyn, and who made an unguarded comment about how awful 'it' was about Sharon. My heart sank.

It wasn't until after her holiday, some hushed whispers and her operation, that Sharon herself told us that she had breast cancer and would need to undergo chemotherapy. It seemed outrageous that positive, strong Sharon should be attacked by something so stealthy and underhand. It was probably the first time any of her colleagues had seen her even close to tears, and most of us wanted to cry with her, but at work you have to hold things together, so we tried not to make it worse. We're a small company, which often feels like a family, and we took it personally.

I was just beginning to feel well again after my own long illness with myasthenia gravis, treatment for which had included major surgery and radiotherapy, and during which Sharon had been amazingly supportive; so this felt like another body blow. I'd hidden a lot of how I felt when I was ill, and I knew Sharon would be even better at it than me, and it was going to be awful. She's also a tremendously stylish woman, and the thought of her losing her hair was heartbreaking.

Typical of Sharon, with her announcement out of the way, she began to talk business again, and initially we stopped her. We wanted to know how she was, and as a fellow mum, I wanted to know how her children were coping. Mine had been very scared by my illness, and Sharon's were a lot younger. Work seemed irrelevant but she insisted we carry on. We felt very protective of her and often wished she would slow down a bit, although realising that work and normality were a practical help. The first morning that she came in wearing her wig, I said, "I thought you were going to have it cut shorter than that." It was that convincing. She looked great throughout, no matter how she felt.

She seemed to take everything in her stride, unstoppably, until John died. This extra tragedy, especially for the children, was too much on top of everything else. It was just before Christmas, and being

Sharon, she still contemplated coming to our work 'do'. At this point two of us took her aside individually and told her to just stop it. Go home and be with your children, we said. Thankfully, she did. She took a month off in the New Year and although we missed her and there seemed to be small vacuum without her, we coped and we were very relieved that she was resting at last.

She returned on form, despite her inability to sleep or taste anything. She was very frank about some of her symptoms, and very discreet about others. You had to piece things together to understand all she'd been through. She also got very matter of fact about the wig - we had an off-site planning meeting at Sharon's house, and the moment we got in she pulled it off. I was struck by how white her re-growing hair was, and how tiny her face looked without her mane - one of Sharon's trade marks, her hair. She looked fragile, almost ethereal, but within a few minutes I'd forgotten about it as we worked on a pitch for a new client - we won the business, snatching it away from a London agency.

Sharon doesn't do half measures; she tackled her illness like all her projects, head on. Watching her through her illness, I occasionally saw the vulnerable side I knew was there, but hadn't often glimpsed. It hasn't done her any harm. I said to her one day, "The trouble with you and me, is we've made it look too easy." Hiding how dreadful you are feeling isn't always the best policy - it doesn't get you as much sympathy or leeway, but there is definitely a place for acting better than you feel, especially at work.

Sharon's illness affected all of us at the time. One or two had to step their game up to compensate and for a while we had little sympathy for wimps. "It feels like you need to have a leg missing before you can have a day off sick," one colleague joked. As time has passed, new people have arrived who never saw her sick, and who wouldn't guess now if they weren't told. Sharon went from being the boss to just being someone we cared about deeply, and back to being both. She can still be a bit larger than life - thank God.

Tina, friend for 30 years
৪৯

The message from Merlyn to tell me the news of Sharon's cancer came as a complete shock but when I spoke to Sharon she sounded her normal positive self and was confident that she would beat it. I have known Sharon for about 30 years, having met at advertising agency Ogilvy & Mather, and remained friends ever since. She has always dealt with everything that life has thrown at her in a very positive way and I knew this would be no different. The first thing I remember her saying was that she was going to get a wig as she was pretty sure that whatever method she tried, her hair would fall out! She knew she was going to have to keep working and couldn't just take time out as many others in her situation could do; she would need to continue to meet clients, so a wig was essential.

Trying to keep everything as normal as possible for the children, plus hold down a full time job, was going to be an enormous challenge but if anyone could achieve this, Sharon could. I had never heard of anyone having chemotherapy sessions at home and was amazed when Sharon told me that was what she had managed to arrange. It would mean that the children would be able to be with her when they came home from school. Sharon has a very close relationship with her sisters and I knew they would all be there to support her but I tried to keep in as regular contact as I could and I know sometimes when I called she was just too tired to talk, but the family kept me up to date with all that was happening.

It is hard to imagine what the children were going through, but Sharon was completely honest with them and explained what was happening with all the treatment, and I know what a huge comfort they were to her. She is a true Mum and I know despite how unwell the drugs made her feel after each session, she just kept going.

When John died so suddenly I thought how much more can the family take? But again, Sharon was there offering support to everyone without a thought for herself. I remember her saying back at the house after the funeral how hot her head was but she didn't want to take her hat off as Richard hated people seeing her bald head.

I have had another close friend who had breast cancer and she also was on her own with young children, but with the support of family and friends coped very well. However, unlike Sharon, she was able to take a year off work, fully paid, and had time to relax between chemo sessions to build up her strength. She told me there was no way she would have been able to work during this period.

Jenny, reflexologist

I first met Sharon towards the end of September. She had had a lumpectomy mid-August, the cancer had not spread into the lymphatic system, but she was suffering with cording on the underside of her arm. She was about to start her chemotherapy treatment and was desperate for complementary support during this period. She had heard that reflexology was a good therapy but couldn't find anyone to treat her. The reflexologists she had approached refused to handle anyone with cancer.

I qualified as a reflexologist in 1995 and went on to study Advanced and Precision Reflexology the following year. My philosophy with my clients is to look after their emotional needs as well as their physical well-being. Reflexology helps to relax the nine body systems, allowing homeostasis (the maintenance of a stable equilibrium) to take place. Sharon was receiving excellent treatment in the tranquillity of her home; my job was to support this and to help ease her way through the invasive chemical onslaught she was receiving.

One day she walked into my clinic (which is run from home so I like to think it is a relaxing environment and not too sterile) looking fabulous but tired. The effects of the treatment had kicked in and lots of symptoms were now leaping up to say "hi". Losing your "crowning glory" is a huge blow to your confidence, but Sharon was blessed with knowing the right people to support her and was introduced to a fabulous shop where she bought an incredibly flattering, spiky wig. It was so wonderful but would drive her crazy when it made her scalp too hot. Walking into my house one day she tore the wig off and the relief on her face was marked. I realised the pressures of maintaining her appearance between home and work was all too much some days, and when her fingernails started to flake off, it was yet another blow to her flagging self esteem. (Patchouli oil and calendula cream are brilliant for this condition.)

These things seem superficial to us outsiders who are not going through a life-threatening course of treatment; we are only too relieved that the person seems to be coping and has an optimistic view of the outcome.

During Sharon's treatment I attended an AOR (Association of Reflexologists) seminar in London on "Reflexology for people with cancer" given by a lady called Edwina Hodkinson. Edwina is a nurse as well as a reflexologist and works at a hospice in Manchester. She had so much advice to pass on to therapists who had not worked with a client with cancer before. Research was presented to confirm that reflexology does not have an adverse effect on a patient having chemotherapy, nor can it override the chemotherapy or make it less effective. "Always work with the person, never the cancer" will remain with me forever.

As Sharon's chemotherapy sessions proceeded, her energy levels seemed to hit an all time low and the need to get to the end of the course of treatment became vital. Poor sleep was a huge issue. In November Sharon had her third session and had felt ok after it. Her fourth session was the day after a session of reflexology; this schedule seemed to help balance her before the invasion of vital chemicals into her body. When I next saw Sharon on the 21st December she told me of the terrible shock of her husband dying so prematurely, at the age of 50, from a heart attack. She was tearful, angry and to add to the pile of emotional stuff going on, she had her fifth session of chemo to deal with. I was exhausted and so sad for her. Watching someone go through such a painful journey would have sent the strongest of families into such a downward spiral, but this was Sharon and her family here, coping in the best way they could, wonderfully well by my observations, but still a tremendous knock back for Sharon.

I work with Chakras (seven energy centres in the body) and practise Crystal Healing. Dowsing over the Chakras gives me a good guide as to where the client is suffering, or out of balance the most. On 21st December Sharon had four of the seven Chakras so out of balance there was no reading at all; so a bit of work there and balance was resumed at the end of the session. Using colours to help heal is a lovely way to do your "homework" on yourself. After all we are the colours of the rainbow; colour influences our lives in so many ways, so why not utilise that energy to aid healing?

Sharon's eighth and final session was on the 22nd February. The skin on the soles of her feet was very dry and peeling. Yet another symptom to deal with. I knew it would pass, but it still had to be dealt with until that time arrived. A month later Sharon was having radiotherapy and her feet were feeling prickly. Oh the importance of how our feet feel! By the time 22nd April arrived Sharon had finished her 20 radiotherapy sessions, her back had locked up that morning which was miserable but, great news, THE HAIR IS GROWING. I've never seen the wig whisked off with such speed. At last, something to get excited about.

Lack of sleep for Sharon was a huge problem, this poor body just needed to rest more. Finding the time to do this between work and home was a big issue. The immediate family were so supportive. Every time I went to Sharon's home to give her treatment there were always visitors: children, sisters, brother-in-law, nephew, the stream of folk was endless. This support and strength would have had a profoundly positive effect on Sharon and her three children.

Phil, oncologist

ℰᕲ

When I first met Sharon I thought that she was probably going to be OK. When you see new patients referred after breast cancer surgery for additional treatment you have to try and weigh them up pretty quickly, even as they walk in and sit down. How frightened are they? How angry are they? Do they look like they are going to trust you? How much do they know? How much do they want to know? Have they been given the right information so far? Has their surfing on the Internet helped or confused them? I could go on.

Sharon gave out the right signals. She was clearly a bit apprehensive as everyone should be when you're about to have a discussion about cancer treatment, but quickly saw that she was composed, intelligent, well informed and funny. She asked the right questions. She smiled. By the time we had finished with each other it was clear to me that she would probably get though the chemotherapy without any major problems. She was someone who dealt with problems, who got on with things.

True to expectation she handled the hair loss, the tiredness, the weight gain, the mouth ulcers, the insomnia pretty well. She accepted them as a necessary evil that comes with the treatment. Every time I saw her during the chemotherapy it was obvious that, although things were unpleasant at times she was easily a match for the treatment, and showed no signs of it really getting her down.

Quite a few women get depressed in the months after chemotherapy has finished. No longer concentrating on getting through the chemotherapy, having to try and get back to "normality" when feeling under par, and worrying about the future can contribute to this. Sharon showed no sign of this happening to her. It was obvious that she had too much to do, too many people to care for to allow this to get on top of her.

How did her cancer affect me she asks?

Having cancer has been repeatedly described as a roller coaster; up one moment and down the next. It can be a roller coaster for the doctor too. In one clinic I may be celebrating the fantastic response to treatment with one patient and then having to break bad news about scan results to a distraught patient half an hour later. I have good days and bad days. However, whether good or bad they are always a bit better after seeing Sharon. She emits this air of positivity that always impresses and, more helpfully to me if I'm having a particularly bad day, she always has something funny to say. Right from when I first met her to now she has always been able to find something humorous about her situation.

The outlook for women who get breast cancer has improved dramatically over the last twenty years, partly as a result of the development of more successful treatments like chemotherapy. Unfortunately this does mean that the treatment to ensure complete eradication of the cancer is more involved, prolonged and often unpleasant.

Sharon is very special but in no way unique. I see many women similar to her. They get breast cancer when they have families to look after and careers to maintain. They take the treatment with guts and determination, continuing to multitask in the way that women can, then come out the other end and get on with their lives.

Nick, Leanne's husband

I'd known Sharon for quite a few years, firstly as her financial adviser, arranging her mortgage and investments and the like but gradually more and more as a friend. I'd come to visit her a few months after she'd been diagnosed with cancer. She'd lost her hair but otherwise seemed fine, she just wanted to get her finances organised and find a way to provide for her children. Her ex-husband John had died quite suddenly only a few weeks earlier and coping with such a loss, plus the treatment, didn't seem fair at all. As bad luck would have it my wife, Leanne, had just been diagnosed with breast cancer too, so we talked about the practicalities of dealing with the treatment, its side effects and our children. It was good to know someone with that degree of recent knowledge and Sharon was as open and honest as possible about everything.

While no one can say chemotherapy is a great experience, Leanne mostly breezed through it as if nothing was going to stop or slow her down; she had a life to live and children to look after and this was not going to stop her. We have three wonderful girls: Victoria now nine, Katherine now seven and Elizabeth now four, and naturally she didn't want them to feel concerned or worried by the treatment so, from the very beginning, we discussed what the cancer was and tried to explain how the treatment would affect her. We even took them all to the hospital at one chemo treatment to show them exactly what happened. The nurses were a little reticent and were not sure about showing them needles going in, but we insisted that it was all or nothing. Like Sharon she had a great wig, so she too never again had bad hair days.

We came to Sharon's 50th birthday celebrations and they had a good old chat about their new curly hairstyles, their own by this time, and what they were doing to lose the weight they'd put on during treatment. It was such a happy time, but it was limited. Shortly after, Leanne starting feeling a pain in her joints, hips I think, so we saw our oncologist (the best oncologist in the UK, Dr Merah). A trip to the hospital and more tests followed to reveal the unthinkable: Leanne's cancer had spread.

Although we thought a mastectomy and removal of the lymph nodes would be enough, it seems that the cancer was more virulent than anyone expected. Scans revealed many 'hot-spots' throughout Leanne's skeleton - hips, spine, ribs, jaw and even the skull. Looking back, that was the point at which we knew that Leanne was going to die… we just didn't know when.

Just how do you tell your children that you are going to die? The answer is you just do, through floods of tears and staccato speech and lots of hugs. The thing is that you realise that you can't hold that level of emotion for any length of time, you soon find that you're not crying, just being practical and making plans and having a cup of tea. The children quite quickly stopped crying, moved on, and were busy involving themselves in other activities - it's the way they deal with stuff like this and, unlike adults, they don't carry the emotion into other areas - must be where men get their tendency to compartmentalise things, because we never grow up! The doctors didn't give up either, and the whole mass of the NHS machine groaned into life as specialists and counsellors appeared from every direction.

Leanne dealt with this as she dealt with everything in life - in her stride. Yes, there was more chemotherapy. At one point her hip broke just twisting round to get out of the car. There was more discomfort, and yes, there were plenty of tears, hers, mine, the children's and everyone else, but Leanne coped magnificently. We made plans for the future, as you must when you have a young family, and treated every day as precious. The future never really seemed to be bleak - even knowing that it was going to be without Leanne, but because our children knew what to expect, we were as prepared as we could be.

I remember that at the very first diagnosis three years previously, we asked her then oncologist what to expect if things were worse than expected, and what the end might be like - he wasn't prepared to even consider the thought and, for that reason, we changed to Dr Merah; we are adults after all, and we felt we needed to know what ALL the eventualities might be.

Leanne's parents live in South Africa, but were quite old now and too frail to travel, so we decided that we should all go there together to enable Leanne to say her goodbyes. Although we had a fantastic time and felt relieved that the visit, which could have been a desperately sad affair, was a happy and loving one, there were only momentary lapses into sadness and, in the spirit of living life to the full, these things need to be done. Wallowing in self-pity was not an option, especially for Leanne.

When we got back to the UK, we carried on as

normal there simply wasn't any other way; Leanne worked with me, so we both went into the office together. Sometimes you could almost forget that there was something wrong, and then you'd remember, and that incredulity would pull you up short. How could such a vibrant, generous, wonderful, young woman be taken from us by something so invisible yet insidious?

Leanne, like me, was angry, furious, sad and disappointed. There was no treatment on this earth that could prolong her life, so together we had to face facts that I, the archetypal hopeless male, would have to become the domestic goddess's understudy.

What was the end like? Horrible actually. In October 2007 we were on holiday in Norfolk and Leanne picked up an infection, the first of many that followed each treatment. She was pretty poorly as we struggled home and I took her straight to the hospital. This turned out to be the point at which her body could no longer fight the cancer, there were just too many tumours and she became weaker with each treatment as the immune system was so depleted. Despite this, she continued to live life to the full and didn't submit to the obvious pain and discomfort she must have felt. I have a picture of us going out to a black tie event in November 2007 and she looks so beautiful you wouldn't know she was dying. We had Christmas together and, on the day before New Year's Eve, we knew another infection had taken hold and we rushed her to hospital again. For the next two weeks the hospital battled to stabilise her and had some limited success. At first she was unable to speak or move but eventually she regained some strength and was able to speak a little - you could see the sparkle was back in her eyes.

But the recovery was to be short lived and things were getting serious. In early January 2008 I had a call to come quickly to the hospital, as they were worried about her condition; she was unresponsive and unable to communicate. After 24 hours of frantic treatment and deep concern, I was advised to gather our children and get ready to say goodbye; this was it. If telling your children that their mother is going to die when she looks well is difficult enough, taking them to the hospital, standing outside the ward and trying to prepare them for their mother's final moments was sheer agony - but it had to be done, and somehow it was. I stayed on overnight and typically she rallied, we even got to the point where she was conscious again and although unable to speak, was able to smile her inimitable smile. But again the seesaw of life tilted the other way and she deteriorated once more. We resolved to try and get her home and hoped she would at least be able to die there surrounded by friends and family. For those of you who may face this in the future, don't be afraid of the implications of someone dying at home, it is by far the most preferable option you can take and although the hospital is geared up for treatment, with the best will in the world it's not a place to die.

Taking advice from the doctors the move home was on and off and on again, as Leanne's condition fluctuated. They thought the journey home would kill her but, as ever, Leanne proved them wrong, she made it home and we had another week in which to share some time together. She was definitely aware of her surroundings at first and she let us know when she was hungry or uncomfortable. The process of death from cancer involves a gradual shutting down of the body's systems and it isn't pleasant to watch a life ebb away, especially one so precious. It was a few short days before she was completely unconscious and the emphasis then was to make sure she was clean and comfortable and in no pain. It's impossible to explain how you know someone who is unconscious is not in pain but you just do; I think it's the expression on the face. You cannot hide from the fact that this is a very unpleasant business - however with superb medical help from the local District Nurses and the endless patience of the night sitters, it was all very dignified - as it should be.

On the 28th January 2008 Leanne's life ended. I

happened to be at her bedside holding her hand - the first time I had had time to just sit and be with her after all the hustle and bustle of the various carers and nurses' comings and goings. The children were at school, Grandma was resting in the lounge and I was reading to her. Then suddenly I noticed that she was no longer breathing.

Strangely the end wasn't what I expected the end to be. There was just a sense of peace and calm and an understanding that she died peacefully in her sleep and this was time for her to leave.

Leanne was a committed Christian; she carried her belief on her sleeve. Her dignity and poise during what was to be her final months on this earth, made me realise that she was very sure of the presence of God in her life and it was her faith that protected her during her illness and would continue to protect her in this life and the next. Regardless of your own belief, Leanne's faith was what gave her her strength, and the knowledge that this earthly end was not the end and, with that, she could leave, knowing that she had done her best for her family and friends.

It's been six months and writing this now is still very difficult, but her faith has given me the inspiration to explore the Christian faith myself and see just what it was that gave her such strength of character. The children continue to grow in all ways and we talk all the time about Mum's death and her life. There are things still to do like organise the memory boxes for the children and go through Leanne's clothes and possessions, but there seems no rush to do this yet. I quite like to look into the cupboards and see her things there; it's comforting in a way. The children are normal and well adjusted (I think) and the fact that they went through the pain and anguish along with her and that we held nothing back, I believe, will make them more rounded, confident individuals. There are still bad moments, rather than days, and that is to be expected. The future will happen whether I want it to or not, so we continue to try and live life a day at a time and as if it's our last - because one day it will be.

Lightning Source UK Ltd.
Milton Keynes UK
177492UK00001B/7/P